Man Against Pain

"And the Lord God caused a deep sleep to fall upon Adam, and he slept: and He took one of his ribs, and closed up the flesh instead thereof;

And the rib, which the Lord God had taken from man, made He a woman, and brought her unto the man."

GENESIS 2:21, 22

Man Against Pain

3,000 Years of Effort to Understand and Relieve Physical Suffering

BERNARD SEEMAN

CHILTON BOOKS

A Division of Chilton Company
Publishers
PHILADELPHIA AND NEW YORK

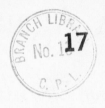

Contents

Man Against Pain

Part I

In the Beginning

Chapter 1

THE BIRTH OF PAIN

All life shrinks from pain. From the simplest living cell to the complex mammal that is man, pain is an experience to be shunned. Where pain cannot be avoided, man and some of the higher animals have learned to ease and even block it.

Man's attempt to conquer pain is older than his effort to hold off death. Pain is an immediate and urgent experience; death is the end of experience. Yet without pain there would have been no life.

An infant reaching out to explore the world would suffer irreparable damage if pain did not mark the limits between safety and danger. He would continue to burn, bruise and cut himself; and his ability to survive would be gravely impaired. The adult, better able to recognize danger, would still be in dire peril without pain's warning signals.

From the beginning, the protective mantle of pain shielded all life. In the turbulence of Earth's youth, an estimated three billion years ago, the first protoplasmic capsules of life that appeared would have been swiftly obliterated if they had not possessed a defensive reaction against deadly changes in that violent environment. Too much heat or cold, the approach of toxic or corrosive substances, too much or too little pressure —any of these could have eliminated the tenuous differences that separated life from non-life.

Actually, how can we define life? Scientists and philosophers have tried to do so for centuries without arriving at a defini-

3

tion that seems to cover all cases. Still, there appears to be general agreement that at least four basic characteristics are necessary to life.

A living thing must be able to take materials from its environment and convert them into energy, heat and the matter of its own substance.

It must be able to grow.

It must be able to reproduce itself.

It must be able to detect and react to stimuli, both internal and external. The reaction to pain is part of this characteristic of life.

Science still knows very little about the mechanisms that regulate these reactions in the living cell. Although it seems to have no nervous system as we know it, the cell must have some means of detecting changes in the environment and receiving a flow of information upon which it can base its "behavior."

Some of this information may indicate the presence of food, and the cell will make the appropriate response. But the approach of something dangerously hot, for instance, will bring a different type of information to the cell's receptors. It will react swiftly, darting away from the oncoming peril. This, in the cell, is the equivalent to man's response to pain.

For countless eons, combinations of chemicals probably crossed and recrossed the barrier that divides life from non-life before one combination appeared that could detect environmental changes and react to them with a protective reflex. With that event pain was born; and life, shrinking from the peril it signaled, was able to survive.

There is a vast span of life stretching from the primal cell to man, yet everywhere within this reach is the inbred ability to sense the warning of possible damage to the organism.

An unusual series of experiments was conducted some years ago by the Indian scientist, Sir Jagadis Chandra Bose, who sought to learn how plants reacted to various kinds of stimulation. Among other things, Bose tested the effects of alcohol, certain poisons, electric currents and even anesthetics. He discovered that the reactions of the plants were fundamentally the same as those of animals, despite the fact that no recognizable nervous structure has been found in plants. After studying the delicate recording devices that measured the results of his work, Bose concluded that "a plant feels pain just as does man, and as do the lower animals." Not only that but plants, like animals, could be anesthetized with chloroform and made insensitive to pain.

The same biological principles seem to work in all living things, and the strongest of these principles is, normally, the preservation of the individual. "Toward this end," wrote Dr. George V. N. Dearborn of Harvard University in 1900, "pain undoubtedly developed, and toward this end pain everywhere, in the long run, tends to work."

Unfortunately, man's understanding of pain has been late in coming and is far from clear. From earliest times, pain was related to magic, to demons and to gods. Only in relatively recent years have we even begun to unravel some of the complexities of the nervous system, and the mechanisms and the pathways of pain. This beginning of knowledge has so far made only minor inroads against the mass of misconceptions —mystical, religious and pseudo-scientific—that has been elaborated over millennia of ignorance.

Pain has been considered a curse or punishment inflicted by some evil demon or punitive deity.

Pain has been considered a test of faith and religious devotion.

Pain has been considered a means of spiritual purification.

Pain has been considered a pathway toward communion with various deities such as Osiris and others who "suffered and died that Man might live."

In savage cultures everywhere, and even in our own, the ability to withstand pain is related to courage, virility or masculinity. And in numerous societies, the rites of initiation into full adulthood frequently involve the infliction of pain which must be endured without flinching.

These and other primitive beliefs that shaped man's attitudes exist to this very day. Perhaps they are not so binding as they were in earlier times, but they still tend to impede our efforts to understand the nature of pain and to find more effective means of alleviating it.

Fortunately for mankind, there were people courageous enough to challenge prevailing attitudes and dogmas, even at the risk of ostracism, imprisonment, torture and death. In the development of the so-called Western civilization, which we cherish for its philosophical emphasis upon humanity, it was frequently deadly to question the sanctity of pain. Only a few centuries ago, people were burned at the stake for seeking to ease the pain of childbirth.

The fact that pain does have its protective uses makes it neither holy nor especially desirable. While skin pain helps provide a quick and immediate response to danger, the value of deep pain is frequently more difficult to explain. This type of pain does have a useful function in providing the initial warning of disease, but after that first warning it frequently serves only to perpetuate the agony.

According to the British physician, Lord Morgan, a person passing out a kidney stone is hardly the better off for doing it in torment. Nor can the victim of a cancer benefit from the pain. In the body's interior, therefore, the mechanism of pain seems crude, ill adapted and relatively without good reason for existence.

The time is long overdue for a reassessment of some of the still-prevailing attitudes that continue to distort our understanding of pain. Pain is neither a force nor a power. It has no being. It is not an object, a punishment, a purifier, nor an event. It is simply an interpretation of information about an event.

You prick your finger on a thorn while plucking a rose.

The penetration of the skin is damaging and may endanger the system. Specialized nerves in the affected area of skin convey this message to the appropriate centers of the brain. There the information is processed and interpreted as an unpleasant sensation, something that pains. Meanwhile, through an emergency circuit known as a reflex arc, you have already pulled back your finger before your consciousness was notified that you had been "hurt."

That, in simple terms, is the pain warning and response system. Roughly, this is all that pain is and all that it is supposed to do.

One of the problems that has muddled our understanding of pain has been the lack of a proper definition. Obviously, if pain is an individual's interpretation of information about an event, it is bound to be subjective. Even if two people receive exactly the same information about an identical event, they are bound to have different interpretations depending upon their backgrounds, their experiences and their prevailing emotional and physical states. Under those circumstances, any attempt to define or measure pain on the level of "feeling" would be meaningless. No two people "feel" pain the same way. What is discomfort to one person may be agony to another. These considerations led Dr. Henry K. Beecher of Harvard Medical School to declare that, "Pain cannot be satisfactorily defined, except as every man defines it introspectively for himself."

Much of the difficulty of defining pain may be due to semantic confusion. The particular problem here seems to arise out of the use of the word "define" to express the concept "describe."

Certainly we cannot describe a toothache in other than subjective terms. "It felt like the devil was driving pitchforks into my jaw," or "It was sheer agony," are statements that may describe how we felt about the toothache. They do not define the toothache so that any other person will be able to know and identify that particular kind and level of pain.

Pain is, after all, an interpretive reaction to a certain class of events that affect the body. Some years ago, Sir Charles S. Sherrington, the noted British neurophysiologist, defined pain as "the psychical adjunct of a protective reflex." This definition may be too spare for those to whom the brevity of science seems barren rather than beautiful. Perhaps we can expand and elaborate it somewhat: Pain is the individualized interpretation of information, transmitted over specialized nerve pathways, regarding events that seem to be damaging to the organism.

From this we may gather something about what pain is and how it is caused. It does not and can not tell us how pain is interpreted by any individual other than ourselves. For that matter, while we can define color, sound, smell, taste and touch, we would certainly find it difficult to know how anyone else "sees" the color red, "smells" the odor of violets or interprets any other sensory information.

When we consider the senses in the light of what is known today, we can see that man actually has more than five senses. Each of the recognized senses, sight, smell, hearing, taste and touch, is a specialized message system that uses specific organs and nerves to bring us only one particular type of information about our environment. Ever since the senses were differentiated, it was assumed that pain stimuli were detected and carried by the receptors and pathways of the sense of touch. This is now known to be false.

The receptors and pathways of pain are separate from those of touch and they carry a different type of information that evokes markedly different interpretations and responses. Pain is, therefore, an independent sense, the sixth; giving us one more than the five with which we usually credit ourselves.

While each of us may interpret or "feel" pain differently, most humans as well as all normal animals and other living things have a similar immediate response—they flinch and attempt to escape whatever causes the pain. This is an automatic, reflexive response that is not under the control of our centers of consciousness. Actually, we react to pain before we even "feel" it.

In man, the pain sense operates on two levels; one of those is primitive and uses primitive reflexes that are below the level of consciousness. The other level, far more refined and sophisticated, uses the higher brain centers which developed much later in our evolutionary history.

The first level of reaction gives us the built-in protective response; the swift shrinking away from pain that enabled the first capsule of life to survive. When we blink our eyes or pull back our hands to avoid pain or injury, we are acting through these reflexes.

The second level of reaction operates through our centers of consciousness. Here we feel the pain, identify it and decide what to do about it. And it is on this level that most of our differences in interpretation and response arise. Here imagination, anticipation and a whole complex of memory associations all act to modulate our particular reaction. Among the many factors brought into play are past experiences with pain, social and cultural attitudes, our personal attitudes, our mood, emotional status, presence or absence of anxieties or tensions, fatigue and the general state of our health.

Pain seems to intensify with fatigue, anxiety, illness, boredom and anticipation. If we worry in advance about the possible pain we will face in the dentist's chair, we actually will feel pain more intensely, and often react more strongly than if we had thought of other things.

Our reflex reactions to pain can be harmful and interfere with attempts to heal our wounds and ease our hurts. The blinking reflex makes it difficult to remove a cinder from our eye. The reflex that makes us pull away from pain could make surgery dangerous if not impossible without anesthesia or some other means of inactivating the pain responses.

Our reactions to pain may differ for strange and inexplicable reasons. In February, 1962, Dr. John S. Lundy of the Veterans Administration Research Hospital in Chicago, declared that people with red hair seem far more sensitive to pain than blonds or brunets, and that brunets are the least sensitive. He also reported that national origin and a person's place of residence seem to influence his ability to withstand pain.

Many other peculiarities about pain have been noted. Protracted pain rarely maintains the same intensity. It tends to wax and wane. Why this should be so is not really known. Scientists suspect that various chemical and mechanical factors in the body may be involved, and that emotional and environmental factors play an important part.

Pain seems to become more intense at night than during the day. This may be because there are fewer distractions at night and more attention is concentrated on the sensations of pain.

The simple act of sitting in a chair can become a painful experience if we concentrate on the sensations we feel in the parts of the body pressing against the chair. But if we read a book, listen to music, engage in conversation or otherwise divert our attention, sitting stops being painful.

Because the pain that protects us can also do us great damage, certain safety devices have been developed through natural selection to prevent us from being overwhelmed by an excess of pain.

When pain comes simultaneously from two or more sources, say a toothache and a burn on the hand, the total pain experienced is not the sum of the two added together. Instead, because the nervous mechanisms involved in interpreting and "feeling" pain cannot divide their attention, the more intense single pain usually monopolizes sensation.

Where an ordinarily pain-producing situation is necessary to survival, it does not seem to cause pain. When a snake's skin is cut or damaged, it experiences pain, but when the snake sheds its skin as part of its normal process of growth, there is no sensation of pain. In a similar way, should we be exposed to pain which is so intense that it might trigger a deadly chain of reactions, we are often shielded by a form of shock that cuts off sensation. What takes place is remarkably similar to what happens when an overload of current makes a fuse blow in an electrical circuit.

There are numerous stories, some quite gruesome, of how normal people have been anesthetized by too much pain. A typical case is that of Reverend E. C. Johnson, who was a British missionary in India a number of years ago. He was attacked by a Bengal tiger and so badly mauled that his arm had to be amputated. He remained conscious throughout the savage attack and, as he later reported, experienced "no pain beyond feeling that my arm was in a vise."

We all know how children caught up in the excitement of play do not feel the pain of their hurts; how athletes and soldiers can be insensitized by the emotional violence of their activities and suffer serious injuries without being aware of them. Emotionally disturbed people are often insensitive to pain. So are people in frenzies of fear, rage or religious ecstasy. Intense emotional experiences seem to dominate the nerve pathways and block out the messages of pain. Fanatics, martyrs, berserks and madmen are able to endure the most excruciating pain and may even seem to enjoy the experience.

Just as there are differences in pain, there are also differences in the mechanisms that carry painful impulses. Surface pain, developed to warn us of external danger, is detected by specialized nerve ends with which our skin and exterior mucosa are amply supplied. We have about three million such pain "feelers" in our skin.

Interior pain is different and has different mechanisms. We cannot shrink away from an inflamed kidney as we can from a hot iron; we have developed no reflex arcs to help us avoid interior pain.

There are also other differences. Cutting, stabbing and so on will cause surface pain, but cutting the interior organs or even the brain, will cause no pain. What does produce pain in the body interior are stretching, distortion, pressure, inflammation and certain chemical reactions. Interior pain can be very intense, yet it is quite different from surface pain, and perceived and communicated by different mechanisms.

Very early man undoubtedly recognized the differences between surface pain and interior pain—but to him the differences must have been magical and demonic. He could see and understand how the stab of a spear, a bruising fall or a sting from a bee could cause him pain. The simple evidence of cause and effect made it obvious. Interior pain was another matter entirely. Its causes were invisible and unknown.

The act of dealing with pain, attempting to avoid, ease or eliminate it, is as old as life itself. When the first living cell flinched from an unpleasant or dangerous environmental change, it was dealing with pain on a reflexive level. And because medicine is, at its very heart, an attempt to ease pain and remove its causes, many of the lower life forms can be said to practice an instinctive form of medicine. Higher on the ladder of consciousness, this act takes on more of the attributes of volition until, with man, a genuine science of medicine is practiced.

A dog, feeling the bite of a flea, scratches to rid himself of both the pain and the flea. A wounded animal will attempt to lessen the pain by licking the wound. A dog with a broken leg will train himself to walk on three legs, relieving the pain and permitting the bone to reset. Monkeys will pluck splinters out of their skin and remove other foreign bodies that cause pain or discomfort. But these are only instances of animals easing their own pains.

Far more significant is the conscious act of easing the pains of others. Here, too, on a primitive scale, man is joined by the beasts. Apes, dogs, horses, elephants and other animals show distress when any of their fellows may be hurt and frequently perform positive acts to ease the suffering and nurse the victim back to health.

With man, the struggle against pain reaches its highest form. The development of scientific medicine and surgery, along with growing understanding of what pain is and how it can be relieved, marks one of the crowning achievements of the human species.

This continuous effort has had no smooth and easy unfolding. Discoverers, explorers and propagators of new ideas, by definition, are men who stand alone. This demands the courage to question, to test and, frequently the most perilous quality of all, to be different. It is a characteristic of any established order, be it tribal, religious, political, social, economic or national, to protect itself by demanding conformity. From earliest times to the present day, the innovator and the non-conformist have been regarded with reserve, suspicion and, often, deadly hostility. Yet they, more than anyone else, have led man out of savagery, given us art, science and civilization and opened the pathway to the stars.

The men who ranged themselves against pain, who sought to learn its nature and its causes, had human weaknesses and human strengths. Some were selfless, others were self-seeking; some were innovators, others were developers; some profited, others were martyrs.

As in all other realms of knowledge, man's exploration of pain followed an irregular route. Discoveries were made and lost, understood and forgotten. In many eras the established order was not prepared to accept or even admit evidence, however demonstrable, that contradicted the prevailing dogmas. In other periods, man's technological and scientific background was not sufficiently developed to accept and cope with new concepts. So, until man became able to balance the various forces that acted upon his development, the tides of knowledge rose and fell along the shores of pain.

Chapter 2

MORE THAN MAGIC

The shambling, two-legged creature who emerged into sapience to become our ancestor was a skilled, highly-critical observer. Relatively weak and fragile, surrounded by creatures swifter, stronger, hungrier and more rapacious, he had to be quick to recognize any sign that portended danger. Even the earth, air and waters were fraught with perils that struck swiftly in the form of earthquakes, storms and floods. So he observed, reacted and survived.

He could also do far more than that. He remembered his observations and related them to other observations. From this came thought and imagination, which he was able to communicate to his fellows and thus begin the foundations of knowledge.

This early food gatherer and hunter had an urgent need to alleviate pain because whatever disturbed or slowed his reactions could be deadly. Fortunately, he did not have to be a scientist to be able to ease his hurts. Knowing nothing of the mechanisms and pathways of pain he nevertheless, by trial and error, by accident and by thoughtful observation, developed a number of primitive but effective ways of dealing with many of his hurts.

A great portion of his pain was caused by obvious events. The fall of a rock could bruise the skin or break a bone. The jab of a thorn, the slash of a sharp stone, the bite of an animal and the sting of an insect all produced pain. So did surface infections and parasitic infestations of the skin.

14

Some of these pains could be relieved almost immediately. The thorn could be plucked out. Other hurts were not as easily cured. Over many generations, however, primitive man found that certain pains could be relieved in a variety of ways.

A hunter with a twisted ankle, forced to wade across an icy stream, may have noticed that the pain was reduced by the cold water. Another might have found that the warming rays of the sun seemed to ease a pain. The application of mud-packs, poultices, the chewing of certain herbs—these and many other procedures gradually found their way into primitive man's armament against the obvious pains. And, it might be added, such procedures had to work in a sufficient number of cases or they would have been discarded.

While many pains could be related to obvious events such as a wound, there was a vast area of pain that had no detectable cause. The pain of internal disease or even headache, stomach-ache, earache or toothache had no detectable explanation. Seeking for direct cause-and-effect relationships, primitive man could only have concluded that where he could detect no obvious cause for a particular event, there must be mysterious, unseen forces at work.

Life for primitive man was, after all, a strange and magical process; and he lived in a fear-infested environment where death reached out at every turn. Not only were the animals and other visible dangers ranged against him, but also the invisible and often implacable world of demons that brought storms, floods, lightning, earthquakes, misfortune, inner pain, weakness, sickness and death.

Early man's theory of disease and inner pain was simple and direct. They were due to the magical intrusion into the body of some object or demon, or by the removal from the body of some vital element essential to life and well-being.

Pain-producing spirits could enter the body through many routes. They could use the skin, the nostrils, the mouth, the ears and, in fact, any body opening. Such beliefs were not confined to the primitives. Even the much later Egyptians, with all their sophistication and relatively well-developed medicine, believed that certain painful afflictions could be caused by the spirits of the dead arriving in darkness and, according to the Berlin Papyrus, "Gliding in the nose backward. . . ." The left nostril was said to be particularly susceptible to this type of painful spirit intrusion.

From the early Stone Age hunters to the Melanesian aborigines of today, spirit and object intrusion has been considered the most important source of pain. This belief is involved in the magical infliction of pain upon an enemy, whether by voodoo, ju-ju or other supernatural technique.

When a doll or effigy of a person is pierced by thorns, the body of the actual person is, by the magic of similars, believed similarly intruded by invisible thorns.

Among the existing Stone Age tribes of New Guinea and Melanesia, the witch doctor or sorcerer is able to cause extreme pain in a victim by what is known as a "ghost shot." The sorcerer uses a special weapon, usually a hollow bamboo tube that is plugged at one end and contains the bones of a dead man. Keeping the open end of the tube covered with his thumb, the witch doctor stalks his victim, aims the tube at him and then uncovers the open end. The ghost of the dead man, imprisoned with the bones, streams out of the tube and into the body of the victim, bringing pain and disease. Rheumatism, arthritis, headaches and other painful ailments are believed to be caused in this way.

Although this type of magical pain-production is, today, mainly confined to the more backward regions of the world, strong evidence exists that it was used in Europe in comparatively recent times. Among the Welsh, lumbago was occasionally referred to as "shot of the elf," and in Germany it has been called "Witch's shot" (*Hexenschuss*).

People still believe in the "evil eye" which can bring pain and misfortune. Some superstitions regarding magical production of pain have become diluted and, although their original meaning is forgotten, are still with us. There was an ancient belief, related to the "ghost shot," that by pointing a finger at a person, painful spirits or a curse could be directed at him. Today, in Borneo and certain primitive parts of the world, pointing a finger at a person is sometimes considered a hostile act that could bring violent reprisal. In the United States and some other Western countries, however, pointing is merely considered to be impolite, although we do not quite seem to know why.

A number of the superstitions regarding magical intrusions have been preserved in our Scriptures. Just as it was known that real arrows and spears cause pain, it was believed that invisible arrows and spears of demons also cause pain. Therefore, inner pain was often attributed to the arrows of an angry or punitive divinity. Job related his own pains to such symbolic arrows when he declared: "For the arrows of the Almighty are within me, the poison whereof drinketh up my spirit. . . ." (Job 6:4).

Unlike the surface pains whose causes were obvious, the magically-caused inner pains, the primitive man believed, required complicated and specialized treatment. Practically anyone could remove a thorn or place a poultice on a bruise, but only a specialist in supernatural arts could lift spells and remove demons or objects that intruded to cause pain. Thus the art of the witch doctor, the medicine man and the priest was born.

These early healers, exercising their powers in the realms of pain and well-being, life and death, were thought to have a wide range of magical forces at their command. They could cast spells and drive them out. They could bring game and plentiful food. They could predict and even influence the future. They could bring success or failure. They could weave spells and enchantments, compound healing or killing formulas, provide magical charms and amulets that warded off demons, diseases, curses and misfortunes. Some were even believed able to arrange for a relatively easy transition into whatever hereafter the particular tribe envisioned. These killers of pain were indeed men of great power and influence and were to become gods, kings and high priests.

The early witch doctors practiced both preventive and curative magic. Certain incantations repeated over a person might make him impervious to pain-producing demons. Charms and amulets could be given such magical force that the person who carried them was provided with a barrier against any evil intrusion.

The preventive magic of the witch doctor found its way into the religious practices that later developed. Incantations became prayers and the magical amulets that warded off evil and pain evolved into holy relics and religious symbols. The dried toad or knotted cord carried by the primitive were believed to serve the same protective purpose as does the crucifix, the mezuzah or, for that matter, the rabbit's foot. Other protective barriers against evil intrusions devised by the primitives consisted of ritual tattooing, wearing earrings, noserings, and necklaces designed and worn to keep evil spirits at bay. These magical practices later came to be considered a form of personal decoration. Similarly, anthropological records indicate that Cro-Magnon man and even the primitive Egyptians rubbed red pastes, powders and juices upon their faces, lips, fingernails and bodies to ward off sickness and pain. Through sympathetic magic, the red symbolized blood, a potent charm that continued the life force. This, too, gradually metamorphosed into a cosmetic practice.

The curative magic of the witch doctor was considerably more complicated than his techniques for preventing pain. First of all, he had to divine the chain of magical or demonic events that had produced the pain or illness, then he had to break that chain at some point so that the intruding demon or object would be compelled to leave the victim.

This could be done by placating the god, the spirit or the sorcerer who had caused the painful intrusion, or by neutralizing the magic that caused the pain with a more powerful countermagic. It could also be done by making things so unpleasant for the intruding demon that he would be forced to flee.

The actual treatment involved placatory sacrifices and the recital of spells, as well as the beating of drums, chants, strange noises, and grotesque dances possibly expected to help scare the demon out of his wits. Magical objects and herbs were burned, infusions of magical herbs were brought to the patient to be smelled, swallowed or rubbed on the afflicted part. The medications consisted of vile tasting herbs and various unwholesome substances such as body excretions. These were designed to disgust the intruding demon and drive him out.

In many cases, pain and illness were alleviated in this way. This argues neither for nor against the method of therapy. After all, the bulk of all human aches and pains will be relieved no matter what sort of treatment is applied or even if they are not treated at all.

On the other hand, the treatment used by the witch doctor was a form of what is now recognized as psychosomatic medicine. While the drugs seem to have acted on physical aspects of the ailment, the incantations, drumming, dancing and other parts of the total treatment managed to affect the emotional components that intensified the pain; relaxing the patient, easing his fears, convincing him of recovery.

Other magical practices came into wide use to relieve pain. It is remarkable how similar they were despite the fact that they came into independent being in widely separated parts of the world at a time when no communication existed. Among the Picts and early Scandinavians, the clothes of a sick person were hung on a magical tree. Through sympathetic magic, the clothing represented the person and carried his symbolic pain. The tree was believed able to absorb the pain and illness, leaving the patient cured. In other parts of the world, if there was a pain in the arm, leg or some other accessible part of the body, that part was tied to a tree which would thereupon absorb the pain.

Among Asian and other primitives, it was believed that a

wooden skewer thrust into the affected part could impale the pain demon. The skewer would then be buried in a deep hole where neither the sun nor moon could penetrate, thus effectively getting rid of the pain.

From ancient into medieval times, people thought that pain demons could be captured and inactivated. They could be burned, fed to cattle, drowned in water or transferred to some other object. The practice of using leeches, still in use in backward parts of Europe and America, stems from the belief that the pain-producing demon is carried in the blood, and that the leech removes the demon along with the blood it sucks. Phlebotomy or bloodletting, one of the most primitive techniques of exorcising demonic invaders of the blood, survived in serious medical practice until relatively modern times. This is a grim testimonial to the inertia of tradition and the power of dogma.

Another medieval practice that survives, fortunately in a more kindly form than originally, is the baking of gingerbread men and other attractive cakes and cookies in human form. Originally, the pain that was "captured" and "removed" from a particular person would be lured into such a cake which was then given to some unsuspecting beggar or passer-by to eat. This might either destroy the demon or transfer him to another host. Today this magical origin of gingerbread men has been largely forgotten, and the traditional cakes are no longer used to convey pain.

The primitive witch doctor was heavily committed to what we deem sorcery and superstition. To him, magic was a tool that helped explain and manipulate events in the world in which he lived. In that very important respect, magic was as valid to him as science is to modern man. What is more, a number of materials and techniques that originated in magical usage, actually became a part of the body of science.

One of the most significant examples of this is in the area of drugs and herbal medications.

In searching for various magical aids to relieve pain, the

primitive doctors undoubtedly sought the help of the spirits which they believed resided in plants, trees, flowers, rocks, minerals and other objects. Gradually, through trial and error, they began to learn that certain herbs, roots, leaves, berries and other substances were helpful in driving off the demons of pain and illness. These were retained in healing practice, and the knowledge was passed down through the ages. The substances that did not help, usually, were quickly discarded.

Out of this combination of magical and empirical medicine a vast body of knowledge regarding the uses and effectiveness of drugs was developed and tested over many thousands of years. Even today, the greater part of the drugs in use have come to us from primitive sources. Opium, India hemp, cocaine, atropine and other narcotic herbs were used by medicine men long before man began to record his history. The American Indians were using the flower of the Jimson weed (*datura stramonium*) to produce twilight sleep far back in pre-Columbian times.

In India, South Africa, among the American Indians and in other parts of the world, infusions of willow bark were used to ease various pains including that which afflicted the joints. This was an early use of salicylic acid, a form of what we now know as aspirin and used for the same purposes. Witch doctors used herbs and other substances as relaxants, anti-spasmodics, laxatives and in other curative functions, including the relief of pain. The modern tranquilizer drugs which have done so much to ease emotional tensions and mental illness were first derived from *rawolfia serpentina*, a herb used for this purpose from ancient times in India.

Early man sought relief from pain everywhere. He found it in many places: in the application of heat and cold, in the use of analgesic drugs, in mud baths and mud packs, in poultices and unguents, in intoxicants and in sleep-producing narcotics. The latter were particularly important in prehistoric surgery.

Even the Dawn man was familiar with certain crude methods of surgery. He could, for instance, set broken bones and learned to perform various operations involving scarification and other ritual mutilations such as circumcision and even castration. Where the operations were done for magical or religious reasons, pain was probably an important part of the ceremony, to be borne without flinching. But in operations designed for healing purposes, various devices, drugs and techniques were used to produce insensitivity, unconsciousness or otherwise relieve the pain.

One of the earliest operations in human history is that of trepanning, opening the skull. According to the records of the fossilized bones dating from Cro-Magnon times, such surgery was performed successfully, perhaps forty-two thousand years ago. They were successful because some skulls show traces of more than one operation, therefore the patient survived at least the first.

Trepanned skulls have been found almost wherever man is known to have existed. They show, among other things, the remarkable similarity in the development of medicine among primitive people who were widely scattered geographically. Not only were similar techniques evolved out of selective trial and error, but they grew out of seemingly similar beliefs.

Headache, an unusually prevalent ailment even to this day, was believed due to the presence of an evil demon in the skull; a theory that seemed to take root in virtually all areas where human life existed. The cure for this was obvious to early man; make the devil leave the victim's head.

The attending witch doctor or sorcerer usually began his treatment with certain spells and incantation. If these ritual exorcisms failed to dislodge the demon from his abode in the victim's skull, then a more drastic treatment was instituted.

As far as can be reconstructed from the evidence of operations performed by the pre-Inca Indians of the Andean highlands, the patient sat with his head held firmly between the knees of the witch doctor who chewed coca leaves, the herb from which the narcotic cocaine is obtained. Using a sharp stone knife as a chisel and a heavier stone as a mallet, the experienced practitioner could work a hole through the skull in a relatively short time. Throughout the course of this operation, he would allow the juices of the coca leaf to drip onto the area of the incision, and this pain-relieving alkaloid would produce an effective degree of local anesthesia. This rather drastic treatment for headaches was not only widely practiced, but had a remarkably high rate of recovery considering the circumstances.

At the very outset of man's emergence as a distinct species, he sought to alleviate pain and suffering. From that day to the present, that quest has continued, evolving along with man himself through empirical trial and error, magic, mysticism and metaphysics until it finally emerged into reason and science.

" Pain-relieving analgesia and surgical anesthesia are no new developments. They were not discovered, as many of us are inclined to believe, by Western man as the outcome of a happy merger of superior Judeo-Christian humanism, European science and American initiative and knowhow. What is new is the refinement, sophistication and controlled use of modern scientific anesthesia, as well as the beginning of an insight into the nature and mechanisms of pain and its relief."

The primitive medicine man was an anesthetist long before the first permanent human settlements were built. Huddled over his smoky fire, he could compound drugs from herbs, roots, seeds, blossoms, berries and leaves, drugs to ease pain, to reduce sensation and even to bring on the artificial sleep of complete anesthesia.

Unfortunately the primitive medicine man left no written record. But the evidence is there in his fossils and his discovered tools and in some of the remarkable rock paintings that have been found in Southern France and in Africa. And more recent, living evidence can be studied in his present-day counterparts, the primitive tribesmen of New Guinea and other remote areas, who have not yet emerged from the Stone Age.

The first trepanning operation took place, as we estimate,

about forty-two thousand years ago. Some thirty-five thousand years were to pass in darkness before man developed the science of record-keeping and thus learned how to write. When that great leap forward was made perhaps seven thousand years ago, as we suspect, by the people of Sumer, our ancestors were provided with a means of compiling, preserving and handing down a record of their discoveries. With that decisive tool man's struggle against pain emerged into history.

Part II

Pioneers Against Pain

Chapter 3

FROM SUMER TO THE PYRAMIDS

When neolithic man learned that he could work the soil to produce food, a profound revolution took place in his activities and attitudes. No longer a nomad, he settled near his crops, founded communities and gained enough leisure to think, to imagine and to invent.

His sophistication increased; and the simple, primitive magic of earlier times was no longer sufficient to help him explain and manipulate this far more complicated world. Now the rains, the seasons, the climate, the birds, the insects, the sun and even the earth itself had to be placated on a regular, cyclical basis. The life, death and rebirth of the crops upon which he depended was elaborated into a concept of life, death, rebirth and afterlife in man. Inevitably, magical practices coalesced into formalized beliefs, rituals and ceremonies, These, in turn, became systematized into religions.

The attempt to understand and treat pain began a strange double development. For the most part it became increasingly involved with superstition and religion. But simultaneously, under the growing pressure of accumulating knowledge and technology, a diverging pathway to understanding was opened, founded on investigation, observation and reason. Of these two approaches, the mystical one remained dominant for many millennia. But the rational method, disdained and frequently suppressed, persisted despite the restraints and ultimately led man toward science.

It is by no means clear when or even where the first civilized communities emerged. The presently available evidence indicates that the earliest settlements, with their developing agriculture and industrial arts, were established in the fertile valleys of the great rivers: the Tigris and Euphrates, the Nile, the Indus, the Hwang Ho and the Yangtze.

Some of the oldest records come from the Mesopotamian plain between the Tigris and Euphrates. There, about seven or eight thousand years ago, a city called Sumer was built by a stocky, dark-haired people who learnt the use of copper and bronze, developed wheeled carts and mathematics, began to chart the heavens and even attempted to calculate the first calendar. But by far the most important gift given us by the people of Sumer was that of record keeping and writing. With this man could begin at last to record and preserve his experiences, thoughts, discoveries and knowledge.

Other cities rose and fell on the Mesopotamian plain which came to be known as Babylonia, cities such as Akkad, Ur and even Babylon itself. In all of these, one of the most urgent tasks that fell to the sorcerer-priests was the relief of sickness and pain. The arts they practiced were largely but not exclusively magical in concept. They used astrology, divination and outright sorcery in their healing, but to this they added a growing knowledge of anatomy, surgery and herbal medicine.

Because of the profound importance attached to the healing arts and the easing of pains, power over these functions was ascribed to specific gods in whose names the priest-physicians acted. Marduk, the Babylonian God of Magicians, was also the god who cured the ills and aches of the people. The priests who called upon his healing intervention used a magical symbolism as treatment; and many of the incantations calling upon Marduk to ease specific pains have been preserved in the clay tablets upon which the Mesopotamians impressed their wedge-shaped writing.

Special demons were identified as being responsible for particular ailments. Toothache was believed caused by the gnawing of a worm, a theory which survived in Europe at least until the eighteenth century. Jaundice was said to be caused by the demon *Axaxazu* "who makes the body yellow and the tongue black."

Significantly, in this ancient statement about a demon, we find the stirring of scientific observation. The medical writers of early Babylonia, despite the fact that they saw the supernatural everywhere, began to make a careful record of disease symptoms and organized their knowledge into rational and accessible form.

One set of clay tablets which has been preserved is divided into three columns. The first column names the disease, the second column prescribes the drug to be used, the third column describes the method of applying the drug. Sorcerers though they were, the physicians of Sumer, Babylon and the developing Mesopotamian civilization were scientifically methodical in their record-keeping.

There is evidence that the early Babylonian physicians advanced a theory that pains in one part of the body might be caused by a center of demonic infestation in another part of the body. This is similar to the modern concept of focal infections. Such a theory was used by King Ashurbanipal's physician. According to the records, he prescribed the pulling of the king's teeth as a treatment for pains elsewhere in the king's body.

One of the first medical gods of ancient Mesopotamia was Sin, God of the Moon. Among his special powers was the rule over the growth and use of medicinal herbs. Because these plants were believed capable of destroying malignant demons, they were used to drive out pain and illness.

In order that the herbs might retain the special power invested in them by the Moon God, they obviously had to be picked, it was ordained, at the time of their greatest strength —when the moon was full. This belief has persisted to the present day, and many practitioners of folk medicine still gather their herbs in "the full of the moon."

How the various herbs were supposed to act to destroy pain

is not at all clear, beyond the fact that they were believed to drive out demons. Yet a number of these medications whose use is preserved in the ancient writings are known to be effective.

About 2250 B.C., a Mesopotamian physician inscribed on a clay tablet a remedy he used to relieve the pain of dental caries. The medication consisted of henbane seeds ground into a powder and mixed with gum mastic. This cement was then applied to the cavity and, in all likelihood, worked quite well.

Two other medications reported in the Mesopotamian writings are worth special mention because they are among man's oldest and most enduring medications. These are the opium poppy and the mandrake, both of which were already considered ancient remedies when Sumer was founded.

Opium and its derivatives are still in use, and the mandrake became important in practically all parts of the world where it was found. The use of this plant undoubtedly began with magic. Because the mandrake root has a somewhat human shape, it was invested with magical power. The early Mesopotamians used the root as a charm against sterility and learned to use it as a specific against pain. This plant, as we now know, has atropine-like properties and, though fallen into disuse, can produce pain relief, sedation and narcotic sleep.

As Babylonian medicine developed out of the early healing of Sumer and Mesopotamia, the practice of surgery achieved growing importance and, what is more significant, an increasing number of lay physicians appeared; healers who were neither priests nor sorcerers.

The Babylonian surgeons, with opium, mandrake and other narcotic and pain-relieving drugs at their disposal, presumably practiced some forms of anesthesia and analgesia to ease the suffering of their patients. Their practices were strictly regulated by a code that emphasized the need for respecting the welfare of the sick.

This code, promulgated by King Hammurabi about 1900 B.C., seems to have been the first recognition by government that a physician had civil responsibilities. The fees that a doctor could charge were clearly listed, and specific penalties were set if the physician failed to achieve a cure.

According to the Code of Hammurabi: "If a physician . . . shall open an abscess with the operating knife and preserve the eye of the patient, he usually shall receive ten shekels of silver. . . ."

But "If a physician . . . shall open an abscess with an operating knife and destroy the eye, his hands shall be cut off."

The surgeon's life could hardly have been a happy one under the circumstances and his use of the knife must certainly have been inhibited. Yet the pressure upon him to learn more and heighten his skills was undoubtedly intensified. His need to gain a better understanding of the structure and functions of various parts of the body was a spur to the study of anatomy and physiology, primitive as these must have been.

At about the time Sumer flourished, another great civilization arose along the silted shores of the Nile. This land of Khem, which came to be known as Egypt, seemed to reverse the process of Mesopotamia. Instead of beginning with a magical approach to pain that gradually tended toward the rational, Egyptian healing was practical and relatively rational at the outset, then declined into sorcery and superstition.

As Egyptian society became more formalized and complex, the growing religious influences brought an increase of mysticism and demonology. Finally, Egyptian healing became smothered in a welter of dogma and ritual.

Healing and the relief of pain were so important to the Egyptians that, as with other early people, these were considered a function of the gods and god-kings. Set, the beast-headed god, was believed to be the divine incarnation of evil who spread pain, disease and plague but who could also cure. The goddess Sekhmet was supposed to have a special power over the pains and ills of women. Thoth, who, it was said, had cured the divine infant Horus of the painful sting of a scorpion, was considered the major healing god of ancient Egypt until he was replaced by Imhotep, who was elevated from mortality to divinity.

Actually all of Egypt's gods were somehow involved in the treatment of disease and the easing of hurts. Ra, the Sun God and Egypt's chief deity, was credited with being the first to use mandrake as a soporific and anesthetic. Significantly, the Egyptians called this plant "the Phallus of the Field" and used it as a charm for potency as well as a specific against pain.

Ra, despite his unimaginable legendary power, was presumably not immune to pain and occasionally required treatment himself. Nor was he above mistakenly selecting an incompetent physician.

One day, according to ancient legend, the Sun God suffered some annoying pains. In looking about for help he decided to call upon the goddess Tefnut who, while not especially skilled as a healer, was noted for her great beauty and charm. Obedient and eager to help, Tefnut prepared a healing concoction which did exactly the opposite. Instead of removing Ra's annoying pain it produced a monumental headache. His agony convinced the Sun God that, in healing at least, skill was more desirable than beauty, so he called upon the goddess Isis. This great enchantress and sorceress, so the story goes on, promptly prepared a remedy that brought an instant cure to Ra's headache.

The formula for this celebrated remedy, preserved in the Ebers Papyrus, is as follows: "Berry of the Coriander, berry of the Poppy plant, wormwood, berry of the Sames plant, berry of the Juniper plant. Make into one, mix with honey and smear therewith. When this remedy is used by him against all illnesses in the head and all sufferings and evils of any sort, he will instantly become well."

Most of our knowledge of early Egyptian healing comes from the writings that have been preserved in the various papyri. One of the most important of these came to light in

1873 and is known as the Ebers Papyrus, after Georg Ebers who obtained it under rather strange circumstances from a mysterious Egyptian.

The Ebers Papyrus once belonged to Pharaoh Amenhotep, who reigned in the sixteenth century before Christ, and is a collection of still earlier medical writings.

This remarkable document reveals how the Egyptians believed in the power of the gods to inflict and relieve pain and disease. One passage, apparently the prayer of a physician, declares:

"He whom the God loves is made alive; I am the one whom the God loves, me he makes alive to pronounce words in the preparations of medicine for all parts of the body of a person who is sick. . . . Isis heal me as she healed Horus of all his pain. . . . Oh, Isis, thou great enchantress, heal me, deliver me . . . from the demonic and mortal diseases and impurities. . . ."

In another part of the papyrus, the physician is told how to treat certain painful ills. "If you examine a person who suffers from pains in the stomach . . . you will say: 'Death has entered into the mouth and has taken its seat there.' You will prepare a remedy composed of the following plants: the stalks of the plant tehua, mint, the red seeds of the plant sechet; and you will have them cooked in beer. You will give it to the sick person to drink . . . and then you will say: 'The disease has gone out from the intestine through the anus.' "

The Egyptian healers became highly skilled in their techniques for relieving pain and disease. Beneath the growing accretion of magical and religious influences, there was considerable sound knowledge about a great number of pharmaceuticals and drugs. Opium, for instance, is mentioned for its narcotic as well as its pain relieving effects.

The Ebers Papyrus contains almost a thousand prescriptions, but, unfortunately, all of their ingredients have not yet been identified. Medicines were used in forms that have come down

present day; pills and suppositories, as well as draughts
ointments. In most cases, their functions were accurately
_____ated to lessen pain.

There were many preparations for the soothing of abrasions,
wounds and inflammations. These were made from various
mucilaginous preparations which seemed to have some pain-
relieving as well as mildly antiseptic actions. There were also
a number of slightly alkaline drugs, quite bland, to be taken
orally for the relief of "pain in the left side" and similar com-
plaints which seem to suggest the pains of peptic ulcer.

Remarkably, a great number of the crude drugs used by these
early Egyptian physicians can be traced down the centuries
through Greek, Roman, Arabic and Medieval times to the
present. With the rise of modern chemistry and pharmacology
in the nineteenth century, many of the ancient drugs were
subjected to intensive testing and a considerable portion of
them were discarded in favor of purified chemicals which
proved more effective and easier to control. Yet, in one form
or another, a large proportion of the medications that relieve
our pains today were prescribed in the name of Isis and the
other healing gods many thousands of years ago by the
Egyptians who left careful records of their use.

There is one Egyptian use of opium that is not recommended
for modern times. This is a prescription used in cases where an
infant cried all night and made it impossible for his mother to
sleep. The remedy consisted of "pods of the poppy plant, fly
dirt which is on the wall. Make into one, strain, and take for
four days."

The wise Egyptians apparently knew that opium was dangerous if given directly to an infant, even a weeping one. So this
remedy was to be taken by the mother who would thus be
enabled to sleep despite the infant's outcries. In any case, the
opium, greatly diluted, would eventually be brought to the
child through the maternal milk.

In addition to using analgesic and narcotic drugs directly

for the relief of pain, the Egyptians were also skilled in surgical anesthesia. Actually their surgery was highly developed, especially in the early times of the Old Kingdom when Imhotep practiced.

The almost incredibly high level of healing at that time, in the third millennium before Christ, is revealed in the *Edwin Smith Surgical Papyrus,* believed to be a later copy of Imhotep's *Secret Book of the Physician.* This papyrus is remarkably free of magical and religous influences and shows a sound knowledge of anatomy and surgical techniques, as well as of specific practices to lessen pain during the operations.

In addition to using opium, mandrake, the fumes of India hemp and other drugs to produce anesthesia, the Egyptians were able to bring artificial sleep to their patients by applying pressure to the carotid arteries of the neck, thus cutting the supply of blood to the brain.

Pressure was also applied to arteries and nerve centers of the arms or legs to produce local anesthesia. This technique is illustrated in a carving discovered on the doorpost of a tomb in Sakkara, dating back to about 2700 B.C. when Imhotep practiced.

The idea of pressure anesthesia seems to date back to prehistoric times and has been widely used throughout history as a means of alleviating suffering and easing the pain of wounds and operations.

This was certainly an empirical discovery. There was then no knowledge of the nervous system or its role in the transmission of sensation. Nor could the primitive physicians have known that interference with the circulation to the brain would produce unconsciousness. But it was clear to them, possibly as a result of some accident that was later supported by the evidence of trial and error, that pressure on certain areas of the body produced loss of sensation, and that pressure on the neck caused unconsciousness.

Later, as knowledge grew and as studies of the nervous

system and the physiology of pain became more productive, the reasons for the effectiveness of pressure began to lose some of their mystery.

The Egyptians, because they embalmed their dead, had a great advantage over other peoples in the study of anatomy. In other lands and under other religions, the cutting open of a corpse was considered a terrible act fraught with the most dangerous consequences. But the Egyptians opened corpses and studied their organs as they prepared them for interment. Still, they did little to investigate the brain and learned virtually nothing of the nervous system. Instead, they believed that the heart and blood vessels performed the functions of the central nervous system and were associated with the sensation of pain.

After the fall of the Old Kingdom, about 2500 B.C., Egypt passed through a period of anarchy during which magical and mystical influences from Asia became increasingly important in shaping Egyptian thought. The strong rational elements in her nascent science and healing arts declined. Tradition and dogma replaced experiment, and sorcery and incantation became the accepted weapons against pain.

The influences that acted upon Egyptian thought were similar in many respects to those that shaped the beliefs of the early Hebrews as well as the more primitive people of the lands bordering on the Eastern Mediterranean. It was commonly accepted among the Hebrews that disease and pain were caused by malignant demons of both sexes. The male demons were called *scadim;* the female, *lilith*. These evil spirits, and there were many of them, were presumed to produce diseases of the throat, asthmatic attacks and a variety of ills, including the intense pain of angina pectoris.

The Hebrews thought the relief of pain and illness could be accomplished by magical and religious intervention. Their prophets believed themselves to be invested with a healing touch when they called upon the Lord for His divine intervention. It was often enough for a prophet to place his hands on the heads of the ailing to bring relief. According to the Hebrews, the prophet Elijah was able to resurrect a dead child through prayer, and the prophet Elisha also resurrected a child and cured a leper in like fashion. As with other peoples, their belief in divine healing, however, did not prevent the Hebrews from also using mundane methods to heal their ills and ease their hurts. The very idea of anesthesia was an ancient one among them and is even a part of their creation myth.

"And the Lord God caused a deep sleep to fall upon Adam, and he slept: and He took one of his ribs, and closed up the flesh instead thereof: And the rib, which the Lord God had taken from man, made He a woman, and brought her unto the man."

So, in Genesis is described the creation of Eve and, since the Creator was mindful of human pain, the first use of surgical anesthesia.

There are many records of the use of anesthetic and pain-relieving drugs by the Judaic people. In performing the symbolic sacrifice of circumcision, a practice dating back to prehistory, they compressed the blood vessels to deaden sensation and thus relieve pain. Opium and mandrake were known to them, and they prepared analgesic unguents which were applied to lacerations and wounds.

In Exodus 30:22–25, when an oil for unction is ordained, the Lord made it very clear to Moses that this should be prepared "after the art of the apothecary. . . ." Apparently, such an art already existed among the Hebrews in those early times.

Although they tended to avoid cutting the human body, certain types of operations were performed. The *Talmud* describes operations for fistula, the treatment for dislocations, Caesarian deliveries and a number of other surgical procedures. Many techniques were used to ease the pain of the patients and, in serious situations, a sleeping potion was administered before the operation began.

This anesthetic drink was probably made of wine mixed with an opiate or with mandrake. It had another strange and peculiarly humanitarian use. When a prisoner faced death by execution, he was given this soporific mixture in order that the pain of his suffering be eased. When used in this fashion, it was called "the potion of the condemned." Some scholars suggest that it was this drink, rather than vinegar, that was offered to Jesus on Calvary, and which He refused.

Chapter 4

FROM THE HWANG HO TO THE INDUS

Like the early civilizations of Mesopotamia and Egypt, those of China and India crystallized around great rivers that nourished their agriculture and commerce. As these people emerged from nomadic tribalism and began to develop the arts and techniques of civilized communal society, they brought with them the accumulated lore and experience that had served them from most primitive times.

As far back as the written records reach, these ancient and fecund people knew and used a wide variety of drugs, herbal and mineral.

To the Chinese, the relief of pain was so compelling a need that healers were usually venerated and sometimes worshipped. Earliest Chinese history is shrouded in legend. Just where mythology ends and history begins is difficult to say, although in recent years archeological findings have confirmed many of the myths as history.

The Emperor Shen Nung, who is said to have reigned about 2700 B.C., came upon the scene relatively late in China's legendary history. He is credited with having taught his people the art of cultivating the soil and the use of agricultural implements. No less important was his gift of the healing herbs. The soil which produced the grains that fed the people, also produced the herbs which could ease their hurts.

An ancient herbal, attributed to this Emperor who came

to be regarded as a major God of Medicine, listed more than a hundred remedies for pain and illness. This was used as a basic text by healers who added their own discoveries. As the centuries passed, the herbal of Shen Nung was enlarged until it filled 52 volumes and became one of the most important works in Chinese medicine.

This book contains more than 2,000 prescriptions and recommends many valid remedies including the use of iron for anemia, mercury for syphilis and opium as a narcotic.

Anesthesia, in China, dates back into prehistory. Opium and mandrake were both used there for this purpose, as were a number of other preparations which have not yet been fully identified.

An unusual use of mandrake by the Chinese, one not related to pain, serves to emphasize the antiquity of seemingly modern discoveries. Hypnotic drugs, such as scopolamine, are commonly used today as so-called truth serums. This "modern" tool of crime detection was used by the Chinese many centuries ago. Suspected criminals were given infusions of mandrake, an alkaloid hypnotic chemically similar to scopolamine. In the resultant state of mental relaxation and confusion, the criminals frequently revealed their guilt.

Surgery was a flourishing art in ancient China. Apart from the operations necessary to preserve life and health, a ritual surgery was practiced to provide the Imperial Court with a vast corps of eunuchs. Because they were deemed less prone to worldly desires and temptations than full men, they were highly trusted and achieved positions of considerable power at court and in the civil service. Consequently many ambitious individuals considered it well worth while to submit to castration, as did a considerable number of status-seeking families who offered their sons to this sacrificial surgery.

The operation was performed by specialists who, according to the records, used anesthetics to ease the pain of their patients.

The exact drugs used are not known, but indications are that they were mainly local anesthetics.

Although a great number of castrations were performed in China, the surgeons were capable of far more complex surgery, some of which required great skill as well as the support of effective anesthetics. Plastic surgery was well known, and operations to correct harelip were frequently and skillfully performed.

So great was the skill of China's surgeons that legends were woven around them. One of these masters, later to be raised to divinity, was Pien Ch'iao who, the legends tell, was even able to transplant organs.

Pien Ch'iao was probably a practicing surgeon some time before the Christian era, although the exact period in which he lived is obscured by mythology. One day, legend has it, he was accosted by a fairy named Chang Sang who gave Ch'iao a precious book filled with wisdom and a package of magical herbs. Ch'iao was instructed to read the book and taste some of the herbs every day for a month, after which he would become a fantastically skilled physician.

Not only did the prediction prove true, but it went beyond Ch'iao's most optimistic expectations. Among other powers, he found that he possessed the ability to see into and through the human body and detect diseases and disturbances of the internal organs. In order to avoid frightening people by making a show of this mysterious talent—an ancient version of modern X ray—Ch'iao pretended to diagnose his patient's ailments by taking their pulse.

One day, says another legend, two men came to him for treatment. He examined them and found that one had a strong will and a weak mind, while the other had a weak will and a strong mind. The account of what followed is supposedly told in the physician's own words by historian Ssu-ma Ch'ien in his biography of Pien Ch'iao entitled *Shih Chi:*

"I gave each of them a subtle drink which reduced them to

unconsciousness for three days. Then I operated on them and explored the areas of the stomach and the heart. I then cut out both the stomach and the heart of each of these two persons and exchanged them between them. So wonderful was the drug that they uttered no sound and, in a few days, I suffered them to return home fully recovered."

The operation described is far beyond the means of present day surgery, and was undoubtedly impossible to even the legendary Pien Ch'iao; but the existence of an effective general anesthetic at that time was well within the realm of possibility. In any case, as the story plainly illustrates, X ray and the painless surgical transplantation of human organs already had a place in fancy if not fact.

Hua T'o was another great physician of China who, like Pien Ch'iao, became mythologized. His skill at easing pain and effecting cures was so great, and his reputation gathered so much luster, that temples were erected to him and he came to be venerated as the God of Surgery. Because of his knowledge of anesthesia, his fame spread to Western lands where physicians and chemists sought to duplicate his pain-relieving potions.

One of the discoveries with which he is credited is an effervescent powder that, when dissolved in wine, was able to produce complete insensibility. Thanks to this anesthetic powder, Hua T'o was held able to open any portion of a patient's body, cut and remove diseased organs, then clean and suture the wound all without the patient's knowledge and without causing any pain.

Unfortunately, neither the powder nor its formula was left for posterity. But the China of Hua T'o already possessed opium, mandrake and other narcotic and analgesic drugs. The smoke of India hemp, too, was used to produce unconsciousness and, in an ancient Chinese manuscript, there is a formula for a hemp mixture which is intended to render a patient insensitive to pain during an operation.

The surgical skill of Hua T'o was soaring indeed. So much so that it was said he could perform difficult operations upon a patient too busy to allow himself to be rendered unconscious.

Something of this sort is supposed to have happened when the hero Quan Kung had his arm amputated. As the amputation began, the brave Kung was involved in a game of skill, one from which the Japanese game of Go is derived. Since the contest had reached a critical stage, Kung would allow nothing to interrupt him. Unable to put his heroic patient to sleep with a general anesthetic, Hua T'o used a most effective local anesthetic and removed the arm while the redoubtable Kung played on. This memorable game, with its accompanying amputation, is immortalized in an ancient Chinese print.

Men are usually greater than the times in which they live. This was especially true of the masterful physicians who defied the incrustations of metaphysics that calcified early science into rigid dogma. Hua T'o was probably one of these, and there were others as well who defied the prevailing taboos in order to help their fellow men surmount pain. At the time Hua T'o is believed to have lived, Chinese humanism had developed to the point where any mutilation of the human body was frowned upon, and a doctor who practiced surgery required considerable courage as well as great skill.

Castration, probably because it was a form of voluntary sacrifice deemed useful to the body politic, does not seem to have come under this restraint. There is a parallel here with Christian humanism which, until relatively recent times, permitted the castration of boys in order that they retain the pure, sweet voices needed to choir praises to the Lord.

From earliest mythological times until the middle of the first millennium of the pre-Christian era, the Chinese appear to have dissected corpses in order to study human anatomy. Then, with the spread of Confucian teachings in the sixth century B.C., the human body came to be considered as something sacred, not to be violated even after death. This cast a great burden on the study of anatomy and physiology, impeding the understanding of the nervous system with its pathways and mechanisms of pain.

Gradually, as philosophy and metaphysics achieved the ascendency over scientific investigation, China's technical capabilities and achievements began to decline.

The Chinese came to believe that perfection existed in the balance and harmony of opposites—the Yang and the Yin. The Yang was masculine, representing heaven, the sun, light, heat, force, hardness, the left side and all positive qualities. The Yin was feminine and represented the earth, moon, cold, damp, the right side, softness and all negative and passive qualities. So long as these opposing principles, which ebbed and flowed in constant interaction, were in equilibrium, all was well. There were peace, tranquillity, health, well-being and the absence of pain. But when the balance between Yang and Yin was upset, pain, disease, disorder and various evils resulted.

It followed from these beliefs that all pain and illness came from a disturbance of the Yang and Yin harmony, and a cure could be achieved by restoring the balance. For instance, if pain was accompanied by a fever, obviously due to an excess of Yang, treatment consisted of either depressing the Yang or stimulating the Yin. A draught to make the patient sweat (moisture being related to Yin) might be prescribed as a means of achieving Yin stimulation. It might also be effective in reducing the fever.

Fortunately, it would have been foolish as well as impossible for the Chinese metaphysicians to discard the practical knowledge and theories gained from earliest times. Instead, they attempted to fit them into the dogma of Yang and Yin. In this way, while adhering to latter-day mysticism, Chinese physicians were still able to utilize empirically-proven methods of treating pain and disease. The prevention of smallpox was a typical example. This disease had been known in China since ancient times and for ages had been kept in check by an inoculation. The crest of a smallpox pustule was crushed into a fine powder which was then dusted into a nostril of the person being inoculated. Like the modern vaccination, this usually produced an immunity. However, in deference to Yang and Yin, the inoculation was made in the left (Yang) nostril of boys, and in the right (Yin) nostril of girls.

The Chinese, although they believed the brain to be merely a form of marrow stored in the skull, did seem to have a concept of some sort of system for the transmission of sensation. However, they believed that this was done through the blood. The actual messenger that carried such impulses was thought to be the pulse.

The physicians of China took the pulse as an essential part of diagnosis. There were three pulses felt for simultaneously, each with a separate finger. Obviously this required a highly selective and sensitive sense of touch. One of the three pulses was called the "inch pulse" and could be used to determine the path of a pain caused by an excess of Yang or heat.

According to an early medical text, the *Nei Ching*, which some scholars claim was written by the legendary Emperor Hwang-ti, "When the inch pulse in the hand is short and without volume, headache results. When the inch pulse within the hand is much too prolonged, extreme pains in the feet and the shinbone result. When the inch pulse within the hand . . . strikes upward, the result is a pain in the shoulder and back."

There were some other curious practices that seem to have originated in China and which have gained some modern credence. These involve the principle of relieving pain and illness through the use of counterirritation. One practice, called acupuncture, treats disease by inserting a needle into the proper part of the body. The other practice, moxibustion, involves the burning on certain points of the body of a woolly substance called moxa, which is prepared from the leaves of wormwood. Moxa burns downward and is removed before it can burn the skin.

According to these practices, which are still in vogue, there are three hundred and sixty-five points on the human body where acupuncture and moxibustion can be applied in order to ease specific aches and ailments. Just what physiological principles may be involved are difficult to determine, although a number of studies are actually under way. However, it appears possible that the nervous system does have a role in these treatments since counterirritation is clearly a factor. The sensation of a particular pain can be reduced by the introduction of other strong sensations.

China, despite the vigorous beginnings of her search for knowledge, slipped into a miasma of dogma and orthodoxy that blocked free investigation and the development of science. This tragedy was not unique to China but repeated itself wherever the early civilizations, and even some later ones, attempted to hold back the torrents of change.

In India, as in China, there were vigorous beginnings and a lusty growth. The conquest of pain was as much a goal of the Indians as of other men. Drugs to relieve pain existed even before the first settlements were built along the Indus. And India hemp or hashish, as well as other drugs that could bring artificial sleep and anesthesia, were in use as far back as memory could reach. In the *Rig-Veda*, the oldest of the sacred books of India, we are told that: "Such herbs came down to us from ancient times, three eras before the Gods were born."

We could conclude that the authors of this great classic of antiquity, said to have been written about 4000 B.C., recognized that man discovered the uses of various healing herbs long before he began to create gods and weave religions. In all, the *Rig-Veda* lists more than a thousand medicinal plants.

The practical healing of primitive times was gradually diluted by magical theories of pain and its origins. The early *Vedas* contain a number of formulas against demons and their human agents. There may possibly have been an interchange of influences between early Indian and Mesopotamian civilizations, but this is not clear from the historical records. However, just as in Mesopotamia, healing and the relief of pain became an important function of the priesthood, although a growing caste of laymen also took up the study and practice of the healing arts.

The Hindu writings attribute the earliest tradition of medical knowledge to the god Indra. Another god, a somewhat minor deity named Dhanvantari, who was physician to the gods, came to be regarded as the chief God of Medicine in India. Unlike other medical deities, such as Imhotep and the Greek Aesculapius who began as humans and were elevated to godhood, Dhanvantari has the unique distinction of starting as a god and being progressively demoted to mortality.

Originally a Cloud God, Dhanvantari received a sacred book from Brahma. This book, the *Ayur-Veda,* or the *Veda of Long Life,* dealt with the various branches of medicine.

As divine physician, he treated the pains and diseases of the gods, then, as time passed, he was reduced in rank to become a manifestation of the god Vishnu. In the later sacred writings, he was relieved of even this aspect of divinity and became a mortal, a king-physician who died of snakebite.

In the earliest period of Brahmin medicine, there was a careful study of anatomy and detailed records were made regarding the bones, muscles, tendons, blood vessels and various organs of the body. This valuable knowledge helped bring about the flowering of Indian medicine that came with Susruta, one of the great physicians of India and possibly one of the greatest surgeons in human history.

Exactly when Susruta practiced is not at all certain. Some historians estimate that he lived during the sixth century B.C., others place him in the eleventh century B.C. One thing is clear, he must have lived before the advent of Buddhism because he made searching anatomical investigations, something which would have been barred to him by the humanism of that gentle creed.

Surgery was a flourishing art in Susruta's time, and with it was practiced an apparently effective anesthesia, both general and local. The removal of tonsils was quite common, as were certain fistula operations and even the excision of tumors. But the surgical genius of early India reached its highest form in the widespread practice of plastic surgery. Only in comparatively modern times has this ancient skill been matched.

There was an interesting if somewhat strange reason for India's plastic surgery. According to the Laws of Manu, which governed the lives of the Indian people, amputation of the nose was a common punishment for adultery and other transgressions. Ear lobes were also amputated for various reasons, and personal revenge frequently took the form of an amputation rather than an outright killing. Since Manu, the Brahmin lawgiver, apparently did not forbid the replacement of a severed member, surgeons had a constant stream of patients who sought to have a nose or ear lobe restored, or some other sort of plastic surgery performed.

With Susruta, who was a great teacher as well as a phenomenal practitioner, these operations became highly refined. Quite naturally, they were done painlessly, under anesthesia. Were this not so, Indian plastic surgery would not have enjoyed the popularity it achieved a thousand years before the Christian era.

The pain-relieving agents used by Susruta and the other Indian surgeons appear to have been narcotics. Wines containing an opiate or other drug were apparently used, as were the fumes of India hemp, hashish. Various analgesic drugs were also known to the Indians, and appear to have been used for the relief of minor aches.

One of the great treasures of the human heritage is the book of surgery written by Susruta. Finally translated into English in 1897 by A. F. R. Hoernle, it reveals a grasp of anatomy that was, for its time, remarkable. Even more, his apparent understanding of public health problems would have been considered advanced as recently as a century ago. One noted passage in his book indicates a relationship between the mosquito and malaria as well as similar fevers. In another passage, he urges that a house be quickly abandoned if the rats behave strangely and die. This suggests that Susruta at least suspected that bubonic plague was spread by rats.

Since India had a rather highly developed industry in Susruta's time, the use of metals was well known, and this permitted the creation of effective surgical tools. In his book, Susruta describes twenty different types of cutting instruments as well as over a hundred blunt instruments. Among these are forceps, cauterizers, knives, syringes, catheters, specula and so on. But the most important instrument, according to Susruta, was the hand of the surgeon.

The surgery and anatomical studies that attained such a great height with Susruta, withered and virtually perished with the coming of the Buddha, who was born about 480 B.C. Mystical considerations regarding the sanctity of the human body, even after death, brought an end to the study of anatomy, so necessary to the understanding and alleviation of pain. In this way an essentially humane creed perversely produced some inhumane consequences.

Science was purged from Indian medicine and replaced by metaphysical concepts involving spiritual purification. The developing systems of Yoga placed great stress upon concentration and on purified states wherein the spirit was released from all physical sensation, including pain. In many respects this resembled the early Christian mysticism which evolved several centuries later.

Pain was universal, according to the Buddha, who attributed it to the frustration of human desires which, in turn, arise out of impressions carried by the senses.

"Birth is attended with pain, decay is painful, disease is painful, death is painful. Union with the unpleasant is painful, and painful is separation from that which is pleasant; and any craving that is not fulfilled, that too is painful . . . and the whole truth concerning the conquest of suffering, lies in the self-conquest which leaves no passion remaining. . . ."

Although they attached predominant importance to spiritual and emotional factors in pain, the Buddhists retained much of the earlier Hindu understanding of the senses. The Indians believed that special ducts radiated in pairs from the heart to different parts of the body, and through these channels were conducted the senses of taste, smell, hearing, vision and touch. This crude version of a nervous system had the heart as its center, completely ignoring the brain.

Gradually, as Buddhism became modified through various sects and cults, it tended increasingly toward purely spiritual concepts. In the Mahayana form of Buddhism that spread from Northern India into Tibet and China, pain came to be regarded merely as an illusion. This conviction arose out of a dialogue between the Buddha and his disciple, Ananda, as recorded in the *Surangama Sutra*. In this sacred writing, the Buddha proves to Ananda that a center for sensory perception cannot exist either inside or outside the body since space, time and all physical phenomena are illusory. Only spiritual perception is a universal and infinite reality. Therefore pain itself is but another illusion from which man may free himself.

Physical pain, which Susruta and the other healers of ancient India had done so much to alleviate, continued to produce its torment despite the metaphysical disputations of the mystics. Infected wounds still ached, angina produced its stabbing agonies and mothers still screamed in childbirth. In the physical world, pain was no illusion.

So, despite Buddhism, Yoga and the other mystical creeds, when King Bhoja, who reigned about 977 A.D., suffered head pains so intense that the Court feared for his life, two physicians, brothers, were called to treat him. Deciding that surgery was required, they administered a drug which they called *sammohini* to induce artificial sleep. Apparently, India's surgeons had not lost the pain-relieving arts of anesthesia which had been practiced in pre-Buddhist times.

The healing brothers opened the King's skull, removed the cause of the complaint, then closed and stitched the wound and applied healing balms. With the operation complete, they administered a drug called *sangivina,* which speeded Bhoja's return to consciousness and reduced the possibility of death. This story is attributed to Pandit Balla in *Anesthetics, Ancient and Modern,* published in London in 1907.

History and legend alike make it evident that the anesthetic and other pain-relieving practices were already old when civilization was still new. This seems to have been true everywhere, wherever man wandered the earth or tilled it. The use of anesthetics is frequently woven into the legends telling of the birth of tribal or national heroes. Because such heroes are usually giants, they are commonly too large to be born in normal fashion.

A typical myth of this sort deals with the birth of the Persian hero, Rustum, a giant who caused his mother grievous pain.

As it happened, Rustum's father, Zal, had been raised on Mount Elbruz by a Griffon; half lion and half eagle. When Zal ventured forth on his own, the Griffon gave him some of her feathers, telling him to burn one whenever he was in extreme need. So it was that when Zal's wife, the Princess Rondabah, could not be delivered of the huge infant Rustum, Zal lit one of the feathers.

Instantly the kindly Griffon appeared and told Zal that he would have to make an incision in Rondabah's side in order to remove his son. But, to alleviate the pain, she also gave Zal an intoxicating drug to administer to the Princess and so make her insensible during the operation. Zal did as he was directed, administering the anesthetic and cutting the hero Rustum out of the body of his mother, who was promptly restored to perfect health.

Chapter 5

THE GREEK REVERSAL—
MYTHOLOGY INTO SCIENCE

Unlike so many other peoples who came out of primitive practicality to build complicated metaphysical systems that confined free inquiry, the Hellenic people somehow reversed the process. With them came an outpouring of inquisitive energy that managed to sweep away restrictive dogmas and reach a dazzling climax in Alexandria.

Exploding out of Central and Western Asia to topple the ancient peoples of the Eastern Mediterranean, these nomadic tribesmen possessed fierce independence and enormous vigor. They never truly allowed themselves to become dominated by religion, but accepted their myths as a form of poetry that offered both guidance and beauty. Yet, to a certain extent, the Greeks did fall captive to various philosophical concepts that sought to explain the universe in terms of harmony, balance and order.

The problem of philosophy versus science, or pure thought versus the results of experiment, was further complicated by another facet of Greek life. As members of a slave society, the free Greeks disdained the products of physical labor, holding them inferior to the results of contemplation. If an experiment involving physical labor contradicted a beautiful concept, the experimental fact was often considered absurd.

Happily, the individualistic Hellenes were able to surmount even this tendency. While some were busy arguing, discussing and building elaborate philosophies designed to explain themselves and their universe in terms of beauty, harmony and perfection, the practical nomadic strain sent others off to search out scientific explanations that could be measured, tested and put to work.

For many generations this dichotomy prevailed, affecting all areas of knowledge including those dealing with the problems of pain. Then there burst upon history Alexander of Macedon, impetuous and impatient, who set the tone of his era when he solved the problem of the Gordian knot by simply cutting it. Thus, for a period, the provable, workable fact became superior to the metaphysical concept, even if that fact disturbed the harmonious balance of some philosophies.

From earliest times, the Greek tribesmen recognized that certain herbs from the earth could ease pain and sorrow, even bring joy. Such drugs were called *nepenthes; ne* meaning negation, and *penthos* meaning sorrow or pain. These and other anesthetic drugs of Greek prehistory were woven into the mythology that carried the seeds of Hellenic science.

The youthful shepherd, Melampus, the first mortal to be endowed with powers of prophecy, was also "the first to devise cures by the use of drugs and purifications," according to the mythological writings of Apollodorus. This came about when he saved some young serpents from death at the hands of slaves who were destroying their nest in a tree.

While Melampus slept, the grateful serpents licked his ears and thus endowed him with special powers which enabled him to understand the languages of birds, beasts and even insects, and to know the healing and pain-relieving properties of herbs.

Greek mythology and Homeric legend are rich in references to pain-relieving drugs, narcotics and anesthetics. When Aphrodite found herself suffering grievous pain, she betook herself to Mount Ida in Crete where she found relief by sleeping in a bed of red poppies. Apparently, even in mythological times, the Greeks knew about opium.

Another pain-relieving herb found on Crete was dittany. This member of the mint family grew on Mounts Ida and Dicte, receiving its name from the latter. Aristotle revived some of the myths about this herb when he wrote in his *History of Animals:* "Wild goats in Crete, when wounded by arrows are said to go in search of ditanny, which is supposed to have the property of ejecting arrows from the body."

The Trojan Aeneas, sorely wounded and in deep pain, was eased by the healing power of dittany, according to Virgil's account of the ancient myth. "Venus, smitten by her son's cruel pain, with a mother's care plucks from Cretan Ida the dittany stalk . . ." From this she makes a brew with which she washes her son's wound. "And suddenly, of a truth, all pain fled from the body, all blood was staunched deep in the wound . . . the arrow fell out, and newborn strength returned . . ."

Mandrake, too, had its place in Greek myth but it was called *circeum*, after the witch Circe who turned men into swine through the use of magical drugs. Because of the mandrake root's likeness to the human form, it was believed to be inhabited by a spirit which could drive out consciousness and which could arouse sexual desire.

According to Homeric legend, Helen was wise in the use of pain-relieving and sleeping-inducing drugs, knowledge which she had apparently derived from the earlier lore of Egypt. "Now elsewhere Helen turned her thoughts, the daughter of Zeus. Straightaway she cast into the wine which they were drinking, a drug to quiet all pain and strife, and to bring forgetfulness of every ill . . . such cunning drugs had the daughter of Zeus, drugs of healing which Polydamna, wife of Thon, had given her, a woman of Egypt."

In the *Iliad*, no less than the *Odyssey*, Homer refers several times to drugs used for the specific purpose of easing pain. When the warrior Eurypylus was wounded, his friend Patroclus, ". . . with a knife cut from his thigh the sharp, piercing arrow, and from the wound with tepid water washed the black blood, and upon it cast a bitter root, which he had rubbed between his hands, a root which slayeth all pain, which stayeth all pangs . . ."

In their efforts to relieve pain, the Greeks found Hypnos a most important and useful deity. God of Sleep, he was the fatherless child of Nyx, ancient Goddess of Night, twin to Thanatos, the personification of Death.

Hypnos was a most welcome god in times of sorrow, sickness and pain. During surgery, his presence was especially desired. Unfortunately, Hypnos slept most of the time and it was difficult to awaken him. Therefore various devices and drugs were used to summon his aid. The Greeks even pretended to believe, and some undoubtedly did believe, that the anesthetic drugs they used did not themselves produce sleep, but served instead to summon Hypnos who granted that boon.

One of the noblest of Grecian myths is that of Aesculapius, who became the God of Medicine and was later merged with Imhotep, the Egyptian physician-turned-God, to become a joint divinity of healing.

According to Homer, Aesculapius was a prince of Thessaly, who had certain healing knowledge and who sired two sons, Podalirius and Machaon, both skilled in medical arts. But Greek mythology tells a more dramatic tale, filled with godly passion, rage and compassion.

One day, Apollo, God of the Sun, surprised a virgin named Coronis bathing in a lake. He became enamored of her, and having spent his desire, went on his way. In due course, Coronis became pregnant, and her father, fearful of shame, quickly married her off to her cousin, Ischus.

When the Raven, Apollo's spy, informed him of the marriage, he flew into a godly rage and sent his arrows to slay Ischus. Meanwhile Artemis, Apollo's huntress sister, let fly with her arrows to kill Coronis. Apollo then descended to earth and, as he viewed the remains of the pregnant Coronis on the funeral pyre, he began to feel pangs of pity for his unborn son. He snatched him alive from the womb and took him to Mount Pelion where he turned him over to Chiron, the Centaur.

Aesculapius grew to manhood under the tutelage of Chiron, the great teacher of Greek heroes, and learned virtually all that could be known of medicine and the healing herbs. He became so adept at his profession that, at the behest of Artemis, he restored to life the dead Hippolytus, son of Theseus and the Queen of Amazons. This invasion of the domain of death so disturbed Plouton, God of the Underworld, that he complained to Zeus, his brother. Zeus thereupon slew Aesculapius with a thunderbolt.

The healing legend of Aesculapius spread and endured. A cult was formed, with many temples and shrines where princes and slaves alike could come to have their pains assuaged and their ailments cured. This cult gathered religious force and endured into the early Christian era.

The preliminary treatment of the sick involved physical and spiritual purification by purging, fasting and prayer. Properly purified, a patient would then be admitted to the *Abaton,* or inner shrine, where he would make an offering and then lie down to await the healing dream, one which usually involved a vision of Aesculapius and his serpent. It was during this dream that the cure, if any, was effected.

It would seem that the dream was probably an hypnotic state, during which the priest-physicians appeared in the guises of the god and his helpers to perform whatever treatment or surgery was deemed necessary. Just how this anesthetic trance was induced is difficult to say for certain. Some investigators suggest that the fumes of a narcotic herb, possibly opium or hashish, were introduced into the Abaton as the patient lay down to await the dream of the healing god.

Throughout Greek mythology and Homeric legend, there was an intensely practical lore of pain-relieving drugs that went side by side with the magic, the poetry and the beauty.

A number of the drugs used by the Greek herbalists were

unrefined versions of alkaloids used today as sedatives and hypnotics. Having no chemistry, the Greeks could not purify their products, extract the active agents or even regulate dosages to maintain a measured level of activity. Nor were these deficiencies unique to the Greeks. They extended into almost modern times and marked the difference between primitive and scientific medication.

Despite their lack of scientific background and techniques, the Greeks did study and experiment with a number of drugs, seeking to learn means of controlling their action. They learned, for instance, that both the poisonous and pain-relieving properties of hemlock leaves varied according to weather, climate and the time at which the leaves were gathered. They knew that this State poison, used against Socrates, could also produce a loss of sensation in the hands and feet which gradually spread inward to the body.

Hippocrates of Cos, the great physician who was born about 459 B.C. and is said to have lived more than a century, used his considerable powers to find effective ways of easing pain. His view of pain was almost modern according to some historians. "Pain is a curse," he is quoted as saying. "Do not believe those Greeks who call it 'the baying watchdog of health.' It is not. I have studied its manifestations and I know that it is not an infallible guide to the seat of disease."

With his disciples, Hippocrates experimented with a number of drugs and techniques. Opium, which could not be controlled too well and which had certain dangerous aspects, was used as an anesthetic but was not found especially satisfactory. Hippocrates is also said to have used cold as a means of producing insensitivity to pain. He would numb a limb by packing it in ice or snow before performing the operation. Today, refrigeration anesthesia or hypothermia is considered one of the more advanced aids to surgery.

The possible use of hemlock as an anesthetic intrigued this great physician who is venerated as the Father of Medicine. Seeking for what he called "the death of pain," Hippocrates believed that "the hemlock, which the great Socrates took . . . that hemlock holds the secret of our search. Notice . . . that it induces sleep and a paralysis of the nether limbs . . . if we could so distill hemlock that we can rid it of its deadly properties, we may find the answer to the riddle . . ."

Greek physicians also knew the ancient art of producing unconsciousness by pressing on the carotid arteries in the neck. As a matter of fact, the very name carotid comes from the Greek word *karoun* which means heavy sleep.

Even Aristotle, though not always a very accurate observer, wrote in his *History of Animals:* "If these veins are pressed externally, men, though not actually choked, become insensible and shut their eyes and fall flat on the ground."

Fortunately, not all pain relief was so drastic. Epicurus, the noted Greek philosopher, reportedly practiced a form of healing which, effective or not, would draw many adherents today. According to Robert Burton, author of *The Anatomy of Melancholy:* "When a sad and sicke patient was brought to him to be cured, He laid him downe . . . crowned him with a garland of sweet-smelling flowers, in a faire perfumed closet delicately set out, and, after a potion or two of good drink, which he administered, he brought in a beautifull young wench that could play upon a lute, sing and dance."

While the Greeks continued to deal with pain on a largely empirical basis, using an increasing number of herbs, drugs and other methods that seemed effective, they had little understanding of the nature of pain. Instead, they speculated on ideal states of being, free from pain and illness, that existed when all elements were in harmony. It was a disturbance of this balance, they said, that brought man his diseases and his agonies. This was curiously similar to the Chinese doctrine of Yang and Yin.

Hippocrates himself, in his book *On the Nature of Man*, stated: "The body of man has in itself blood, phlegm, yellow bile and black bile; these make up the nature of his body, and through these he feels pain or enjoys health . . . pain is felt when one of these elements is in defect or excess, or is isolated in the body, without being compounded with all the others . . ."

This rather odd view of pain was typical of the times and arose out of the philosophic concept of the humours rather than from scientific observation and experiment.

Plato, for his part, believed that pain resulted from the violent intrusion into the body of the four elements that made up the universe: earth, air, fire and water. Such an invasion, he explained, caused violent and irrational movements of the soul.

Fortunately, while many Greeks spun elaborate theories, a few were willing to risk the degradation of labor in their search for truth. One of these early scientists was Alcmaeon of Croton, a city of southern Italy, who was born about 500 B.C.

Alcmaeon was unique because he is believed to be the first Westerner to study anatomy by actually dissecting and examining the corpses of animals. Some of his findings were of vast importance and originality, even though they contradicted a number of prevailing philosophical notions. One of the most striking of his observations was that the brain and not the heart was the seat of sensation as well as of motion, and that sleep was produced by certain events in the brain.

This was a revolutionary concept, far in advance of its time, and one that laid a basis for the recognition and investigation of the nervous system. Plato must have noted Alcmaeon's theory because, in his *Phaedo*, he declares through the mouth of the dying Socrates: "The brain furnishes the sensations of hearing, sight and smelling, from which memory and judgment are born, and from these sensations, once established, wisdom also is born."

All this seems to have been disregarded by Aristotle, whose observations, when he made them, were frequently colored by his philosophical expectations. So, more than a hundred years after Alcmaeon began the preliminary exploration of the nervous system and the pathways of pain, Aristotle saw the brain as a sort of sponge that served as a cooling apparatus, and wrote of the heart and blood vessels as the instruments of sensation.

Centuries later, after the works of Aristotle had been given the force of dogma by the Church, these notions were to retard the study of the nervous system for almost a thousand years.

While Aristotle ranged and sometimes stumbled over the whole field of knowledge, some of his pupils became notable specialists. Among these was Theophrastus, who was born on the isle of Lesbos about 370 B.C. A meticulous observer and annotator, he has been called the first scientific botanist.

From his writings it would appear that the mandrake was one of the most widely used plants among the Greeks. "The leaf of the mandrake, they say, is useful for wounds, and the root . . . when scraped and steeped in vinegar . . . for sleeplessness and love potions."

Altogether, in two great works which contained fifteen books, Theophrastus carefully described and discussed all of the known plants, combining both ancient lore and his own studies. His achievement, one of man's great scientific landmarks, stood as the classic work in its field for almost 2,000 years.

When Aristotle left the Lyceum in Athens, he arranged for Theophrastus, whom he cherished, to teach there as his successor. Aristotle, meanwhile, went on to teach another notable pupil, Alexander of Macedon.

It was in Alexandria, capital of the Egyptian fragment of the vast domain which crumbled with Alexander's death, that the Hellenic genius reached its scientific pinnacle. Under the rule of Ptolemy I, one of Alexander's Macedonian generals, Alexandria became the world's first intellectual capital, a meeting place and crossroads of ideas and knowledge such as never before existed.

To this great city came artists and artisans, poets and physicians, metaphysicians and mathematicians. Ptolemy, a man of extraordinary intellectual gifts, set up a Library and a Museum where all the world's available knowledge was gathered and translated into Greek.

At the Alexandrian University, where the most brilliant men of the period came to work and exchange ideas, the fullest freedom of thought and experiment was encouraged. It was truly a golden age of the creative spirit, not to be matched again until the Renaissance.

From the scientific standpoint, the intellectual promise of Greece reached its fulfillment in Alexandria. New attitudes had been introduced by Alexander. The products of labor and experiment were no longer held inferior to the products of pure thought. If a fact could be demonstrated it was no longer discarded simply because it contradicted some metaphysical abstraction.

In the endless struggle against pain, the great need from the beginning has been for a scientific understanding of its nature, how it is perceived and transmitted, how it can be blocked. This required, for a beginning, a detailed study of the structure of the body and the functions of its organs.

Alcmaeon had already begun to dissect animals to study their anatomy, with some notable discoveries resulting. But humans differed in many respects from sheep, goats and dogs. True, human dissections had been performed in China prior to Confucius, in pre-Buddhist India and by the more ancient Egyptians, but religious and other considerations had made this impossible in Greece. The Greeks believed, for instance, that a human did not end his mortal existence with death, but with burial. Therefore, to open a human cadaver was akin to murder.

It is indeed ironic how, throughout most of our history, anatomical studies that could have advanced knowledge and eased suffering were objected to on humanistic, religious and legal grounds which held the dead human body too sacred to be opened. Yet throughout this period, without any comparable outcry, live human bodies were being mangled, shredded, burned, tortured and otherwise uselessly destroyed in executions, wars, religious disputes and other controversies.

In Alexandria, fortunately, this strangely aberrant double standard was briefly put aside. The first of the great Alexandrian physicians was Herophilus, a grandson of Aristotle, who was born in Chalcedon, a city of Asia Minor, about 330 B.C. After studying in the medical school at Cos, he was attracted to Alexandria by the scientific freedom allowed under Ptolemy.

Believing that the human body possessed unique qualities which differentiated it from other animals, he told Ptolemy that a meaningful study of human anatomy could only come through dissections. Ptolemy found this reasonable.

Bodies of executed criminals were brought to Herophilus and, it is said, he began a school of anatomy, performing many of his dissections in view of his students. His courage in violating the ancient taboo, later made him a target of considerable calumny. Grisly fictions were manufactured and, centuries later, he was called "Herophilus the Butcher." In the second century of the Christian era, the Church father, Tertullian, accused Herophilus of having dissected 600 living people while Ptolemy watched with sadistic delight.

Regardless of the misrepresentation and distortion that were turned against him, as they were against so many who dared to challenge entrenched superstition or dogma, the value of Herophilus's contributions is beyond question. He made a systematic study of the anatomy of the brain and spinal cord. He made a clear statement of the fact that the brain was the central organ of the nervous system, supporting Alcmaeon and contradicting the statements of Aristotle.

Herophilus must indeed have been a remarkably acute investigator. Using the limited instruments of the time, he was able to show the difference between the nerves and the blood vessels, something that was very vague in the voluminous Hippocratic writings. He was also the first to note that the brain was divided into different sections, distinguishing the major frontal section, the cerebrum, from the smaller cerebellum. Then he went on to trace the course of nerves from the brain and spinal cord, recognizing them as being involved in movement and sensation. With this unusually original work, man took a long step toward his ultimate understanding of the nature and pathways of pain.

The intellectual freedom of Alexandria was a magnet that attracted the most brilliant minds of the age. Hero came, the maker of the first steam engine; Archimedes, who organized the basic laws of mechanics; Eratosthenes, who knew the world was round and measured its diameter with an error of only fifty miles; Hipparchus, who mapped the stars; and Euclid, who constructed a system of geometry.

Just as this heady atmosphere of Alexandria drew Herophilus, it was bound to exercise its attraction on Erasistratus, who arrived about a generation later. Although born on the island of Cheos, this physician and scientist was raised in Antioch, capital of the Selucid Empire, another fragment of Alexander's shattered domain. He had traveled widely, studied in many schools, learned that many conflicting theories existed and that tradition was no guarantor of truth.

Shunning dogma and preconceptions, Erasistratus seized upon the freedom to study and experiment, to test and prove each theory before he would accept it. In the course of his monumental work he traced one of the most nearly accurate maps of the circulatory system that had been drawn up to his time. No less important were Erasistratus' study of the brain and nervous system and his investigation of the anatomy of the brain in normal and in abnormal states.

Erasistratus maintained that each organ in the body is supplied with arteries, veins and nerves; the arteries and veins carrying blood, the nerves transmitting impulses to and from the brain. He even recognized and distinguished between nerves involved in movement and nerves carrying impulses of sensation. This fact was noted in the first century writings of Rufus of Ephesus, who also attributed to Herophilus the belief that the nerves of voluntary movement originate in the brain and spinal cord.

Another physician of the first century, the Roman, Celsus, drew particular attention to the interest the two great Alexandrians had in the problem of pain. In a deeper sense, Celsus was pleading for the need to revive the study of human anatomy, which had once more fallen under the restraints of superstition.

"Moreover, as pain and also various kinds of diseases arise in the internal parts, they hold that no one can apply remedies for these who are ignorant of the parts themselves: hence it becomes necessary to lay open the bodies of the dead and to scrutinize their viscera and intestines . . . for when pain occurs internally, it is not possible for one to learn what hurts the patient unless he has acquainted himself with the position of each organ or intestine; nor can a diseased portion of the body be treated by one who does not know what that part is."

Erasistratus, suffering from an incurable disease, ended his life with poison on the island of Samos about 250 B.C. This was then a common practice among the infirm. After his death, the intellectual climate of Alexandria gradually went into a decline. Waves of superstition and dogma rose once more and, aided by wars and other calamities, eroded and swept away the triumphs that had marked this creative release of the human spirit. Even the Library, one of mankind's great treasures, was finally destroyed by fire in the third century, when Diocletian put down an uprising against Rome. But, thanks to the Greeks and especially the Alexandrians, pathways had been opened to the study of anatomy and physiology: weapons essential for the conquest of pain.

Chapter 6

"... THEY CALL THE ROMANS BARBARIANS"

The uniform, precisely-marching legions of Rome swept away the bickering remnants of Greek power and brought order, organization and conformity to the world. An intensely practical people, the Romans believed in doing rather than in thinking; they were more interested in visible results than in invisible theories. The early Romans, like other warlike people, considered pain a test of virility and masculinity, but even among them pain came to be a problem with which they had to deal. A man in agony is not at his most efficient, either as a soldier or administrator. And the Romans valued efficiency. At first, however, any intellectual approach to medicine was distrusted; too much theorizing, philosophizing and experimenting were considered somehow unmasculine, effete and not Roman.

Their attitude toward the refinements of Greek medicine is strongly expressed in a letter written by Cato to his son Marcus. Warned the defender of ancient Roman customs and manly virtues:

"The Greeks are a hard and perverse race. Believe me when I tell you that each time this nation brings us some new knowledge, it will corrupt Rome; but it will be much worse if it sends us its physicians; they have sworn to kill all the barbarians by means of drugs, and they call the Romans barbarians. Remember that I forbid physicians to you."

In spite of the opposition of this outspoken senator, who staunchly believed that cabbages could cure many ills and pains, the gifts of Greek medicine did spread to Rome and many of the physicians of the Empire were either Greek or Greek influenced.

The Romans, of course, had their ancient herbal lore which dated from mythological times. A vast armament of plants and drugs existed that, accompanied with the proper incantations or prayers, could ease pain or summon sleep. Lucina, the Goddess of Childbirth, aided by certain drugs, was capable of "pouring an insensibility to pain down all the limbs of a woman in the throes of labor."

One of Rome's ancient sedatives was a bitter, milky juice derived from the mature lettuce plant. This was called *lactucarium* and came to be widely used to induce calm. The virtues of the lettuce were recognized in the chronicle of the tragic love of Venus and Adonis. "After the death of Adonis, Venus threw herself on a bed of lettuces to lull her grief and to still her desires . . ."

Galen, the Greek physician who became one of Rome's most noted healers and who sought to organize medicine into an infallible system, was particularly fond of lettuce. Shunning strong narcotic drugs, he recommended lettuce and, in his later years, came to use it himself. Whenever he could not sleep, or when his mind was overexcited or stimulated, he ate liberally of lettuce and "a soothing slumber" overtook him.

During the first century of the Christian era, the knowledge of pain-relieving and other drugs was summed up in *De Artibus*, the encyclopedic work of Aulus Cornelius Celsus, who was, without doubt, one of the most brilliant men of classical times. In the medical section of his work, written about 35 A.D., he preserves and illuminates much of the earlier knowledge, including the work of the Alexandrians.

"For producing sleep," wrote Celsus, "the following are good: poppy, lettuce, mostly the summer kind in which the stalk is very milky, the mulberry, the leek."

Regardless of their cultural attitudes and heroic poses regarding pain, the Romans normally sought whatever help they could find in alleviating it. This led to a device, attributed to Celsus, that was used well into medieval times for producing surgical anesthesia. Known as the soporific sponge, it was made by impregnating a sponge with the juices of various narcotic herbs and tying it over the patient's mouth. With its fluids being slowly swallowed and its fumes inhaled, the soporific sponge was apparently able to make amputations bearable. According to some historians, even cancerous breasts were painlessly removed.

Like most good physicians, Celsus knew that drugs, while useful, could also have harmful effects and should therefore be used with care. "Pills are very numerous and made for various purposes. Those which relieve pain through sleep are called anodynes; unless there is overwhelming necessity it is improper to use them; for they are composed of medicaments which are very active and alien to the stomach."

These anodyne pills, whose formulas he then provided, were composed of such drugs as opium, henbane and mandrake. Celsus even recommended a pillow, stuffed with mandrake fruit, as a means of inducing sleep and treating insomnia.

The use of this seemingly ubiquitous plant was described in some detail by another noted physician, Pedacius Dioscorides, a Greek surgeon who served in Nero's army between the years 54 and 68 A.D.

"One cyathous (1½ ounces) of the wine of mandrake is given to those who cannot sleep, and such as are in grievous pain, and those to be cut or cauterized, when it is wished to produce insensibility to pain."

His service as a military surgeon gave Dioscorides vast experience in dealing with pain, something that proved particularly useful in his preparation of *De Universa Medicina,* a book that was used by physicians well into the sixteenth century. In this book, he assembled all of the pharmacological and medical knowledge of the time, undoubtedly dipping heavily into the records of such earlier writers as Theophrastus. He described the medicinal use of some 600 plants as well as animal substances and minerals, including some which had never before been mentioned as remedies.

It is clear from his and other writings that the use of anesthetic and pain relieving drugs was an accepted feature of the medicine of that day. Dioscorides calls opium "a pain easer and a sleep causer." He suggests mandrake for local as well as general anesthesia, recommending the use of *morion*, the white seeds of mandrake, in a number of his preparations.

From the vantage point of modern knowledge, it would be natural for us to question just how effective these early anesthetics actually were. Britain's Sir Benjamin Ward Richardson asked himself that very question while he was investigating the anesthetic properties of various drugs during the nineteenth century. Because the directions recorded by Dioscorides were so clear, Sir Benjamin compounded one of these prescriptions and swallowed it. Afterward he reported: "The phenomena repeated themselves in all faithfulness, and there can be no doubt that in the absence of our now more convenient anesthetics, *morion* might still be used with some measure of efficacy for general anesthesia."

While the Romans may not have been great scientists and innovators, they were solidly practical in their medicine. Surgery without anesthesia would have been most difficult so, since anesthesia was available, they used it. Roman medical literature indicates a far more general and scientific use of pain-relieving drugs than was permitted in Christian Europe more than a thousand years later.

Apuleius wrote in his second century book on herbs, "If anyone is to have a limb cut, cauterized or amputated, he may drink half an ounce of mandragora with wine; and while he sleeps the member may be cut off without pain or sense."

Numerous drugs were also discussed by the naturalist Pliny the Elder, a contemporary of Dioscorides. His remarks about hemlock are especially interesting. "Hemlock, too, is a poisonous plant, rendered odious by its use by the Athenian people as an instrument of capital punishment . . . however, as it is employed for many useful purposes, it must not be omitted." Pliny then mentions the use of the hemlock as a poultice to allay eye pains.

Even Galen, who systemized classical medicine and whose work, like Aristotle's, was to be stamped with the authority of dogma by the Christian Church, used various anesthetics in his surgery. But this fine physician recognized that the drugs then in use were extremely powerful, not well controlled and frequently dangerous. "I abhor, more than anybody, sleep producing drugs," he declared, avoiding their use except where he thought it essential.

Accumulating knowledge, more precise techniques and skilled observations made it possible for men like Galen to detect and examine many things that had previously gone unnoticed. This peculiar characteristic is common to scientists and had been possessed by such men as Alcmaeon, Erasistratus and Herophilus.

Physicians of the time had begun to notice that while opium put a patient to sleep and made it possible to operate without pain, the effects were not always uniform. Sometimes the patient died, seemingly from the opium itself. Mandrake, alcohol, henbane, hemlock and other drugs seemed to work differently at different times and on different patients. Sometimes they did little to ease pain, sometimes they produced coma and death.

Other anesthetic techniques were also unpredictable and therefore dangerous. The Romans, like many more ancient peoples, used manipulative anesthesia—pressure on the carotid arteries—to induce unconsciousness. But if the flow of blood to the brain was stopped an instant too long, paralysis and even death would result.

Galen, and others like him, were aware of the dangers and, being unable to cope with them, sought to avoid them. Primitive anesthesia had reached its highest point. The trial and error methods of empirical medicine could go no further. It was no longer enough to know that certain drugs seemed to work for some mysterious reasons. Instead, there was much more that had to be known.

What was it in a drug that worked? Could this be extracted and purified? Could a drug be made that had uniform strength so that a specific dose would always have the same effect? How did these drugs act and why did they sometimes fail? How did they block pain? How did they produce unconsciousness? What was pain? And what was consciousness? At Galen's time, in the second century of the Christian era, these questions could be asked but the answers remained far off. There was, as yet, no scientific chemistry capable of analyzing, extracting and purifying the active substances of drugs. Nor was there any way of knowing how drugs worked without first having a firm basis of anatomy, physiology, neurology and a whole series of sciences that had yet to be born.

So, at the time the Roman Empire entered its period of decline, the struggle against pain stood at a new threshold; one that might, had man crossed it, have led him swiftly into the next period of scientific development. But the tides of history turned him back and man was to wait almost fifteen centuries before he could finally step across this threshold of knowledge.

Part III

The Tide of Pain Returns

Chapter 7

THE FLIGHT OF KNOWLEDGE

Rome was long past her zenith when, in the second and third centuries after Christ, a series of devastating plagues swept across the lands of the Mediterranean. Smallpox, bubonic and typhus ravaged the world that had been enclosed by the Roman eagles, taking an incredible toll of many millions of lives. There were locusts and famine, economic devastation and revolt, all adding unbearable stress to the crumbling fabric of what had once been a vast and orderly domain.

Beset by disaster, the political, social and economic organization of Rome fell apart and the remnants were swept away by the massive migrations of Germanic tribes from the north and the Hunnic peoples out of the Asian steppes.

Confused, wracked by hunger, poverty, disease and chaos, the people of the Mediterranean basin seized at almost any straw which offered hope. Increasingly, they turned for salvation to the Messianic creeds that flourished in the decaying wreckage of Rome. The despairing, the hungry, the sick and the poor, seemingly shorn of all hope, found enormous emotional attraction in almost any promise of salvation that demanded only faith.

Of the vast number of cults and faiths that sprang up, four became so powerful that any one of them might have achieved absolute dominance. There was the worship of Mithras, God of Light, who attracted the slaves, the impoverished and the downtrodden with the promise of immortality.

73

His special day, Sun-day, was later adopted by the Christians, as was the plentiful burning of candles in religious ceremonies.

The Seraphic faith taught that their god was a savior and leader of souls who could raise the dead and bring salvation to all who believed in him. The communicants of this religion worshipped not only the aspects of Seraphis, the Father, and Horus, the Son, but also the Mother Isis as she held the divine infant, Horus. Combining a number of earlier faiths, the mysteries of this Trinity exercised a vast attraction and had a considerable influence on later Christian theology.

Another religion that won a great following arose out of the healing cult of Aesculapius. To the communicants who worshipped him, this medical deity became Aesculapius the Savior who could ease men's burden of pain and sorrow.

The fourth faith, Christianity, directing its first appeal to multitudes of slaves, poor and oppressed, taught that Jesus could heal all ills of the spirit as well as the flesh, and would bring salvation from all worldly evils and oppressions. This faith rapidly spread its appeal to other groups and became the most potent of all. By the fourth century it had largely replaced the other three religions. Aesculapian shrines were razed, and the statues of the healing god were occasionally hauled to the Christian temples where they were set up and worshipped as representations of Christ, who took upon himself the pain and suffering of mankind.

The promise of Christianity was so attractive and asked so little that it rapidly became one of the most powerful and best organized forces in the Mediterranean world. Its inner discipline and cohesion cut through the boundaries of nation, race and class. This was clearly appreciated by Constantine the Great who, hoping to use it as a binding force to establish unity in a world of turmoil, officially recognized Christianity in 313.

In order to prevent differences of theological opinion from creating disputes which might be reflected in the political arena, Constantine convened the Council of Nicaea in 325.

There, where the Church fathers even exchanged blows, according to the account of Bishop Eusebius, the stormy meeting finally endorsed the Holy Trinity and the divinity of Christ, rejecting the various minority views as heresies to be rooted out and destroyed. There could be only one Truth, just as there could be only one Emperor, and whoever questioned this was doomed.

Christianity spread out rapidly from the Mediterranean hub, carrying its gentle preaching along with its dogmas which brooked neither competition nor contradiction. Consequently all of the earlier teachings, those of the Egyptians, Greeks and Romans, were rejected as pagan falsehoods. Scientific investigation, experiment, even philosophic questioning were forbidden since these were a challenge to the dogma of faith that represented the ultimate truth beyond reason or evidence.

At one stroke all the knowledge that had been won over the millennia, the science, the developing arts of healing and pain relief were excommunicated. What need was there for science in the face of miracles worked by faith? And what need was there for drugs, for surgery or for anodynes and anesthetics when faith was the medicine that could heal all ills, banish all pains and even raise the dead?

The medical techniques of the early Christian healers were rooted in the Epistle of St. James: "Is any sick among you? Let him call for the elders of the church; and let them pray over him, anointing him with oil in the name of the Lord.

"And the prayer of faith shall save the sick, and the Lord shall raise him up . . ." (James 5:14, 15)

The attitudes of the early Christians toward pain were shaped by theology as well as by the martyrdom many had suffered at the hands of the Romans. Jesus, himself, had undergone the agony of the Crucifixion and this pain, suffered that man might be redeemed, was touched with divinity.

If pain could redeem, it could also purify. Borne with faith, it could bring man into communion with the Lord who had suffered on the Cross. Thus many of the martyrs had faced their tortures with equanimity and even anticipation, shielded by the anesthetic self-hypnosis of intense devotion. And a number, no doubt, actually sought out pain as a means of purifying themselves of sin and proving the quality of their faith. Pain became so charged with mysticism that the cross itself, an ancient and widely used instrument of torture and execution, became an object of veneration and blessing.

Suffering became associated with piety and even with spiritual beauty. These attitudes regarding pain prevailed for many centuries and exist among us to this very day. There are many religious sects, the Flagellantes of Mexico to name only one of the more extreme groups, who scourge themselves as an act of faith. This neurotic compulsion toward pain and self-punishment is not confined to any one religious group. Hindu and Islamic fanatics are but two examples of many.

Despite their mystical attitudes toward pain, the Christian healers placed great value upon life and the human spirit. Jesus was the gentle healer of the flesh as well as the soul and His followers were enjoined to attempt to follow in His steps, sacrificing themselves, if necessary, to ease the hurts and sufferings of others.

In the turmoil of the times, with war, pestilence and famine taking a hideous toll, care of the sick and the suffering was a matter of deep religious concern. Sanctuaries were set up where the ailing could come for help. These were under control of monastic orders and the medicine they practiced combined the theories of St. James with earlier practices of exorcism. Pain was attributed to demons and evil spirits and could be conquered by prayer, by faith and by the intervention of special saints. The relics of these healing saints—a bone or perhaps a lock of hair—were believed potent aids to a cure. But the medicine of Galen, of Hippocrates and of the brilliant Alexandrians was condemned and cast aside as pagan falsehood. So, with the triumphant spread of Christian humanism over the Western world, science was replaced by Revelation and dogma became unassailable truth.

That a portion of the human heritage of knowledge managed to survive can be related, paradoxically, to the completeness of the triumph of Christian orthodoxy. Nestorius, the venerable Patriarch of Constantinople, had held that the divine and human natures of Christ were separate and that Mary was therefore not "the Mother of God." Like other heresies, this could not be tolerated and Nestorius and his adherents fled into exile.

They settled in Egypt, Persia, Syria, India and some even found their way into China. In the tolerant Orient they were permitted to set up their churches, to worship and to teach. Fortunately, they brought with them much of the accumulated learning that had been extirpated by the defenders of dogma. The Nestorians had salvaged books of Aristotle, Hippocrates, Galen and others who had enriched human understanding. These books were translated into the languages of the lands that gave sanctuary to the Nestorian exiles.

The Nestorians were encouraged to set up schools in Syria, Mesopotamia and other Eastern countries where they taught philosophy, science, medicine and other learning that had come out of classical antiquity. The healing arts were preserved and the drugs and techniques for the relief of pain remained alive in man's knowledge. In this way, what remained of Western knowledge survived and was then enriched by the intellectual explosion that came with Mohammed and the spread of Islam.

The Islamic faith was simple, direct and taught a brotherly equality that exercised great appeal. Strictly monotheistic, it had no established church and no clergy as such, each man being expected to be able to read and understand the *Koran*. This placed a broad emphasis on literacy and, with this, came the spread of Arabic as a common language throughout the world of Islam.

With this new faith came a veneration for knowledge and learning. This is best expressed in the Islamic teaching which holds: "Science lights the path to Paradise. Take ye knowledge even from the lips of an infidel. The ink of the scholar is more holy than the blood of the martyr."

During the early centuries of Islam, while the Christian world rejected or destroyed whatever was not endorsed by dogma, great universities were built in the Arab world. Supported by the state, they became centers of learning which, like Alexandria, welcomed men of all faiths, nations and races who could contribute to the precious store of knowledge. Among the physicians and healers who flourished under Islam were Africans and Indians, as well as Nestorian Christians. But the greater contributions seem to have been made by the Jews and the Arabs.

Judaic medicine, which reached great heights under Islam, had a rather curious development. In the Jewish theological scheme of things, God was the Divine Healer and, consequently, there was scant theoretical need for physicians. However, wounds did have to be bathed and broken bones had to be set so the Jews, a practical people, were able to reconcile the need for worldly medical aid with the belief that God was the only true healer. Advised the *Talmud*, the collected books of Jewish law, wisdom and commentary: "One should call upon a competent doctor and with all his heart hope for the help of Heaven."

To the Jewish physician, every human being in pain was deserving of treatment, be he Jew or non-Jew. Anyone who suffered was an ailing vessel of God to be healed if it were at all within the power of prayer and medicine. In Deuteronomy 23:7 it was declared: "Thou shalt not abhor an Edomite; for he is thy brother: thou shalt not abhor an Egyptian; because thou wast a stranger in his land."

The medicine practiced by the Talmudic healers throughout the world of Islam was largely rational and highly effective. They were skilled in the use of drugs for the relief of pain, were competent surgeons and excellent observers. The *Talmud* apparently recognized that the brain was more than a mere mass of marrow-like material. Instead, it declared that "The seat of reason is located in the skull." There are also some indications that the Jewish healers may have recognized the existence of the central nervous system and some of the functions of the spinal cord in transmitting impulses of sensation and movement.

While most of the medical advice in the *Talmud* was rational, a few lapses did occur. One was a headache cure effected by cutting the throat of a wild rooster with a coin of pure silver and letting the blood flow on the aching part of the head. The blood, it was believed, would wash away the pain. Fortunately, the skilled Jewish healers were likely to disregard such vestiges of magical pain relief.

Science flourished under the encouragement of the Arabs, and chemistry, as distinct from alchemy, began to take on genuinely scientific characteristics. This was particularly important because of the effect it was to have in the preparation of pain-relieving drugs.

In earlier times, medications and drugs had been unreliable because there was no uniform means of preparing or even testing them. Consequently it was a lucky healer who could predict with any accuracy what the effects of a medication would be twice in a row. But with the Arabs, chemistry and pharmacology developed to a point where drugs became more uniform than before and were more likely to have a predictable effect.

It is said that the great Arab skills in making pharmaceutical preparations arose out of the important cosmetics industry. In Persia, particularly, the preparations of perfumes and cosmetic coloring materials had long been an almost precise science. The fragrances and tints had to be virtually exact each time they were prepared. Out of this experience in serving the demands of beauty came the precision and uniformity which helped establish a dependable science of pharmacy. A number of Arab and Jewish physicians became highly skilled in this developing science of drug preparation which did so much to aid man in his conquest of pain.

One of the great early chemists, known as Gerber, lived during the seventh century and is said to have discovered mercuric chloride. Another fine chemist and possibly one of the greatest physicians of Islam's period of medical supremacy was a man known as Rhazes, a Persian born in 865. An excellent musician as well as physician, he is credited with being the first to use sutures of animal gut for the repair of abdominal wounds, something which was supposedly suggested to him by the lute strings he knew so well.

Among a vast number of other contributions, we also owe to Rhazes the technique of distilling alcohol from starch and, reportedly, the discovery of sulphuric acid. Both of these were of immeasurable importance in many areas of technical development, especially in man's struggle against pain because they were later used to prepare ether.

Persia seemed the motherland of Islamic physicians. One of the greatest of these, and his genius reached into many fields, was Ibn Sina, known to the Western world as Avicenna. Born in Bokhara in 980, he studied the *Koran* which he knew perfectly at the age of ten, then turned his intellect to philosophy, astronomy, geometry and, finally, medicine.

With the works of the Greeks and Romans available to him, thanks to the Nestorians, Avicenna studied and elaborated upon them, finally codifying his knowledge into a major work, the *Canon* of Avicenna. In its five volumes, the *Canon* dealt with many matters, disease, diagnosis, treatments, public health, epidemics and surgery. In the fourth volume there was a section devoted to cosmetics. In the fifth volume he described, in meticulous detail, the preparation of healing and pain-relieving drugs.

Avicenna's understanding of pain came largely from Hippocrates, Galen and Aristotle. He believed that "pain is a sensation produced by something that is contrary to the course of nature," and went on to enumerate fifteen types of pain. Among these were corrosive, boring, stabbing, throbbing, compressing, itching and tearing pain.

For the relief of pain there were three groups of substances that could be used, according to the *Canon.* There were those which are contrary to the cause of pain, those which are generally soothing and may cause euphoria or anesthesia, those which dull the sensations in the painful parts. The drugs recommended ranged all the way from healing poultices to narcotics. Avicenna recommended that, where possible, the physician should attempt to remove the cause of pain. But, "if it is desirable to get a person unconscious quickly or to procure a deeply unconscious state so as to enable pain to be borne . . ." he suggested the use of opium, henbane or mandrake preparations.

Many other Islamic physicians and scientists contributed to preserving and expanding the heritage of classical knowledge during its exile from Christian Europe.

The eminent botanist, Ibn Al-Baitar, who was born in Malaga, Spain, in 1197, prepared one of the most complete books on medical herbs. Called the *Corpus of Simples,* it combined the earlier works of Dioscorides and Galen with original discoveries by Al-Baitar. Of the more than 1,400 drugs described in this book, some 330 were noted for the first time.

Not long thereafter, Al-Kahun-Al-Israeli, a Jewish pharmacist of Cairo, wrote a book which came to be considered one of the best texts on the art and science of drug preparation. This book enumerated many herbs and simples, gave clear directions for their gathering, preservation and preparation into drugs and, most important of all, set up standards for the profession of pharmacy.

The beginning of scientific drug preparation that came with the Arabs had an impact on Europe even before the Crusades brought the West into clashing contact with Islam. For centuries, one of the richest sources of profit for the merchants of Venice and Genoa had been the justly famed Arabic drugs contained in cylindrical jars of Persian and Moorish design. Later, through copying these jars, the Italians were able to make the beautifully glazed pottery known as faience ware.

Fortunately, not all healing knowledge had been driven from Europe during the early Christian period. Neither prayer nor faith could banish all pains. Some were so intense that they simply could not be borne, therefore earthly intervention and medicine became necessary. In some parts of Europe, magical and miraculous medicine was widely practiced. Sometimes, as in primitive times, the magic was combined with a rational treatment.

Among the Saxons of the British Isles, who had inherited some of the medical knowledge of the Druids, henbane was used to relieve the pain of pregnancy. But, because the pain was believed caused by a demon that had to be driven away, the henbane, combined with other herbs, was burned beside the woman and, as she breathed the smoke, the following charm was intoned: "Keep away pain of the abdomen, keep away pain of the head, keep away pain of the back."

The incantations could not have been very effective but the henbane fumes may have had a pain-relieving action. In other parts of Europe, candles and prayers were offered up to particular saints to cure specific pains. Without the support of rational treatment, prayers were less likely to be helpful.

The rational healers who remained in Europe must have been dedicated and courageous men since they practiced under the dire threat of heresy. Most of them seem to have found their way into the Church where they were able to function with some degree of protection.

One of these was Hilary, a Christian convert of the fourth century who was elected Bishop of his native city of Poitiers. While writing on the Trinity, he made a number of significant side references to anesthesia. He even distinguished between loss of sensation due to disease and anesthesia resulting from drugs. ". . . and if through some disease a limb becomes withered, it loses the feeling of living flesh; it can be cut or burned, it feels no pain whatsoever because the soul is no longer mingled with it.

"Also when, through some grave necessity, part of the body must be cut away, the soul can be lulled to sleep by drugs which overcome the pain and produce in the mind a deathlike forgetfulness of its power of sense. Then limbs can be cut off without pain, then flesh is dead to all feeling and does not heed the deep thrust of the knife because the soul within it is asleep."

Bishop Hilary, apparently, had available medical knowledge of earlier times. Similar knowledge was preserved or hidden away in a number of the monasteries which had become sanctuaries where the sick came to have their ailments healed and their pains assuaged.

There were a number of these healing monastic orders and, within their sheltered walls, the dogmatic medicine prescribed by St. James was often supported by a growing practice of rational medicine.

One such monastery was founded near Squillace by Cassiodorus. Another, which was unfortunately destroyed by bombardment during World War II after the Nazis had converted it into a seemingly impregnable stronghold, was the Benedictine Monastery at Monte Cassino.

Actually, the monastery had been built on the site of a Temple of Apollo which was itself razed by St. Benedict of Nursia who founded the order which received his name.

In these and a few other sanctuaries, some of the ancient manuscripts were preserved and studied by the monks. Thus they retained an inkling of the medications and healing practices that had been developed by the so-called pagans of earlier civilized times.

Possibly as a result of the fact that they had some knowledge of rational medicine to draw upon, the Benedictine healers of Monte Cassino won the reputation of being able to perform miraculous cures. The afflicted who could make the journey came from all parts of the Christian world to undergo treatments which, strangely, seem to have been patterned after those provided in the shrines of the healing god, Aesculapius.

Typical was the case of King Henry II of Bavaria, as reported by Pope Victor III, who, in the eleventh century, wrote four books describing the "medical miracles" of St. Benedict. Suffering from kidney stones which caused him intense pain, King Henry went to the monastery to seek relief. There, after placing himself in the hands of the healing monks, he passed into a deep sleep and saw a vision of St. Benedict who came and operated upon him, removed the stones and placed them in his hand.

The event was identical to similar events that supposedly took place in the earlier shrines, except that this time St. Benedict, rather than Aesculapius, came during the healing dream.

In all likelihood, King Henry did go to Monte Cassino and did have some stones removed. This operation had been well known to the Romans and Greeks and had already been old in Susruta's time more than a thousand years before. What is interesting in Pope Victor's account is the indication that some form of anesthesia was used by the Benedictines. It has been suggested that the monks used opium or hashish to send their patients off to sleep. Other medical historians speculate that the anesthesia was effected by the use of either mandrake or a soporific sponge similar to that developed by Celsus, permitting the operation to be performed without pain. There is evidence that a soporific sponge may indeed have been used since a formula for such a sponge exists in a Monte Cassino codex that dates back to the ninth century.

The formula for a similar sponge was described by Nicholas of Salerno in his *Antidotarium*, written during the twelfth century.

"Take of . . . opium, juice of hyoscyamine, unripened berry of the blackberry, lettuce seed, juice of hemlock, mandrake, ivy . . . put these all together into a vessel and plunge therein a new sea sponge just as it comes from the sea, taking care that fresh water does not touch it. Then put this sponge in the sun during the dog days until all the liquid is evaporated. And when there is need, dip it a little in water not too warm, apply it to the nostrils of the patient and he will quickly go to sleep. When you want to awaken him, apply juice from the root of the fennel and he will soon bestir himself."

Therefore, as Christian Europe, too, began to bestir itself and rise out of the Dark Ages, the struggle against pain started to regain some of its lost vigor.

Chapter 8

BY THE GATHERING LIGHT

Knowledge may be imprisoned or destroyed but human curiosity, the urge to know, cannot be blotted out forever. For more than a thousand years during the Dark Ages, scientific learning was suppressed but, inexorably, the restraints had to wear thin.

Man's environment changed, new nations and kingdoms came into being. The clash of cultures that came with the Crusades prodded Europe with the attraction of other ways and strange knowledge. New needs developed and new social pressures emerged. Trade grew and expanded along with a greater exchange of information. All this combined to weaken the barriers of dogma that had been raised against knowledge. Inevitably the vast heritage of classical science that had been held in trust by the Arabs and Jews, who had extended and enriched it with their own contributions, started to filter back.

In Spain, the Islamic world with its great libraries, universities and cultural institutions rubbed shoulders with the gaunt Christian world, counterpoising science against mysticism, learning against blessed ignorance. Brave individuals, spurred by the same restless curiosity which had lured man out of the caves, rose to the challenge.

One of these was Constantine of Carthage, a physician who spent many years traveling and studying in Arab lands. He returned to the West and, after serious difficulties with certain of the devout who sought to kill him for consorting with the heathen, he retired to Monte Cassino. There he spent his remaining years translating many of the Greek and Roman classics from Arabic into Latin.

In Spain, the Islamic city of Toledo gave up its treasures to the Europeans under Alfonso VI of Castile. Among the most precious of them were the Arabic versions of many of the works of Aristotle, Euclid, Hippocrates and Galen. A noted scholar of the period, Gerard of Cremona, learned Arabic so that these books could be rendered into Latin.

Although this was ancient knowledge, to the Europeans emerging from a long darkness it seemed to have the glitter and excitement of new discovery. Suddenly they saw a host of new weapons against pain, many drugs, narcotics and techniques that might succeed where even faith failed.

All this was vital knowledge that would help hold back the tides of pain. But it was not yet a step forward. Rather it was a reconquest of the past and not a very complete one. Thousands of years of treatment by trial and error had shown which drugs eased pain and which did not. But this had no relation to an understanding of the nature of pain or how it was perceived, transmitted and interpreted.

Some preliminary explorations of the nervous system had been made by the Chinese, the Hindus, Alcmaeon and the Alexandrians, but this knowledge still had to be regained and could certainly not be confirmed or extended without the freedom to question, to experiment and to study the anatomy and physiology of the human body. All this, of course, remained forbidden. Furthermore, even if the restraints were lifted and the physical nature of man could again be explored, new tools and technologies would have to be developed, as well as new sciences.

The microscope that could make nerve cells visible was hundreds of years in the future. Before such time, there would have to be an optical industry capable of grinding lenses. A refined chemistry and biochemistry as well as a knowledge of electricity would have to evolve before one could begin to trace how the nerves transmitted sensations of pain and other impulses. And the functions of circulation and respiration would have to be known before a science of anesthesia could be developed that was relatively safe and predictable. Man had much lost ground to make up and, when it had been regained, he would still be barely past the beginning.

The first steps that could be taken, even under the rigid restrictions imposed by dogma, were in the study of anatomy. The dissection of the human cadaver had been forbidden since early Alexandrian times. Even the physicians of Islam had been unable to extend their knowledge of anatomy because the human body, containing the soul, was considered too sacred to be mutilated except in punishment or war. However, surgery was practiced and, where a surgeon may not have known anatomy to start with, he frequently was able to learn as he continued to work. Each operation, after all, was a lesson in anatomy.

In medieval Europe, surgeons learned as they operated and, in due course, combined their knowledge and passed it on to their apprentices and students. At Salerno in Italy, the first important medical school of the Christian era was established during the early Middle Ages. This school possessed an invaluable source which attracted students from all parts of Europe—the books that Constantine of Carthage had translated from Arabic into Latin.

Then, in 1240, a set of rigid standards for the teaching of medicine was decreed by Emperor Frederic II. For the first time in Italy, there was set up a system of organized medical study that established a pattern for other universities which sprang up throughout Europe.

Anatomy, at Salerno, was studied by the dissection of pigs and other animals. By and large, nothing new was really learned about the human anatomy and nervous system because the major emphasis was on interpreting and studying the ancient Greek texts, using rare animal dissections to confirm rather than to test Galen and Aristotle, whose work had finally been given the authority of dogma by the church. Yet, at Salerno, a basis was laid for the next advance in man's struggle against pain.

With the Church gradually relinquishing its hold on the practice and teaching of medicine, students at such medieval universities as Bologna and Montpellier pressed forward to enlarge the field of study permitted them. Oddly, because these schools did not have elaborate establishments for the study of anatomy, lectures were often held in taverns and brothels. The books used were those of Galen, Avicenna, Aristotle, Rhazes and other classics. As translations from the Arabic continued, the remarkable herbal works of Dioscorides and others became available.

So, while a scientific study of anatomy was preparing to come into being, the knowledge of the ancient drugs and techniques used for the relief of pain rapidly spread over Europe.

Hugh of Lucca, one of Christendom's most distinguished physicians of the thirteenth century, had served with the Crusaders in Syria and Egypt where he learned advanced surgical techniques. He is credited with using the soporific sponge and other methods to produce both general and local anesthesia. Hugh's son, Friar Theodoric of Lucca, who became Bishop of Cervia, was also a noted surgeon credited with using narcotics and other anesthetics to alleviate pain.

In England, the medieval surgeon, John of Arderne, used both local and general anesthetics. To produce sleep, he usually gave his patients opium or henbane in wine. Frequently, he found, this caused too deep a sleep, so he cautioned his students: ". . . and know that it is well to tweak the nose, to pinch the cheeks or to pluck the beard of such a sleeper to quicken his spirits lest he sleep too deeply."

One of the most famous surgeons of the Middle Ages, Guy de Chauliac of France, whose book *Chirurgia Magna* became the standard work on the subject and paved the way for the French barber-surgeon Ambroise Paré (who is known as the father of modern surgery), urged the use of narcotic fumes as a form of inhalation anesthesia.

Actually, the use of anesthesia became so common during the Middle Ages that it found a place in the literature of the era. In his *Decameron,* Boccaccio tells in the tenth story of the fourth day how the surgeon Della Montagna refused to operate without an anesthetic on a patient with a gangrened leg. "The doctor was of the opinion that without an opiate the man could not endure the pain . . ." Therefore the good doctor "distilled that morning a type of water after his own composition which had the faculty of bringing to the person who drank it sleep for as long as was deemed necessary to complete the operation."

Sleep-producing drugs also came to be used for purposes somewhat less high-minded than the relief of pain, according to a number of romantic tales of the Middle Ages. In the *Knight's Tale,* Chaucer wrote:

> "For he had given his guard a drink so
> Mixed of spice and honey and certain wine
> And Theban opiate and anodyne,
> That all that night, although a man might shake
> This jailer, he slept on and could not wake . . ."

Nor were anesthetics the only means used to ease pain and improve an ailing person's condition. The thirteenth century French surgeon, Henri de Mondeville, was not above psychological trickery. When he had a patient whose state seemed particularly bad, he might forge a letter to him telling of the death of an enemy. If the patient were a priest, the doctor might send him a letter announcing that he had been raised to bishop. De Mondeville, a most realistic physician who saw medicine as a career rather than a calling, advised other doctors to refuse to take on difficult cases wherever possible and never to interfere with desperate ones.

Despite the return of rational medicine to Europe and the stirrings of experiment and study, the influences of theology and the fear of heresy continued to exercise their stultifying effect. This was especially true in the areas of pain relief since, as religious doctrine held, the Lord had ordained pain to be the lot of mankind. Thus any attempt to alleviate pain was frequently considered an effort to block God's will.

Some, who mixed strange brews to ease pain, were considered in league with the devil, and were burned as witches and warlocks. Others, courageous enough to seek out corpses upon which to make forbidden anatomical studies, were held in superstitious dread as ghouls to be swiftly destroyed.

So, with attempts at science often considered witchcraft, theologically-acceptable magic carried the force of truth and science. This resulted in a number of curious practices.

Since Christian Kings were believed to rule by divine right, they held some of the powers of divinity and were therefore able to cure by the laying on of hands. Edward III of England, merely by touching a patient, was belived to cure scrofula, then known as "the King's Evil."

In the sixteenth century, when Henry of Navarre triumphantly entered Paris, the sick lined the streets as he approached the palace. He descended from his carriage and went from one to another, moving his thumb and forefinger over the painful area in the sign of the cross. As he made the vertical movement he said: "The King touches thee." With the horizontal movement he declared: "God heals thee."

Thus Henry proceeded to the palace.

Faith and religious relics were also considered effective instruments against pain. In France, the remains of St. Margaret the Virgin, martyred at Antioch in 303, were held vastly more precious than the crown jewels. Whenever a French queen went into labor, the remains of St. Margaret were brought to the lying-in chamber where they were supposed to assure a safe and painless delivery.

Even faith without the aid of relics or the laying on of hands could protect the body from pain, according to the medieval schoolmen. Wrote St. Thomas Aquinas: "The blessed delight that comes from the contemplation of divine things suffices to reduce bodily pain."

Even where some useful drugs were given for the relief of pain, a number of curious magical practices remained associated with them. Mandrake, that strange root of ancient times, remained one of the most widely used of medieval anodynes. It was still believed that the mandrake was somehow semi-alive, that it possessed human qualities and even sex. The male mandrake was supposed to be white while the female was a deep black.

Gathering the mandrake was a perilous occupation because, unless proper precautions were observed, the screams of the root as it was torn in agony from the earth could drive the hearer mad. To preserve their sanity, or even their lives, medieval mandrake hunters were advised by an ancient herbal to: "Stuff the ears with good beeswax. Then sift the earth around the mandrake and tie one end of a long piece of string to it. Attach the other end of the string to a dog's tail and give a sharp kick in the wretched cur's loins. As the creature jumps forward, the root will give its dreadful cry and the dog instead of the man will go mad or drop dead."

In this strange dual world of magical religiosity and emerging reason, men still found the courage to seek out and to test truth. One of the scientific pathfinders of the thirteenth century was the Spanish physician and alchemist-turned-chemist, Raymond Lullus, who had undoubtedly been inspired by the chemistry of Islam. One day, working with sulphuric acid and other substances, he produced a colorless fluid which seemed to have rather peculiar properties and which he named "sweet vitriol." Nothing much came of this experiment, although the results were recorded. Unrecognized at the time because man's scientific development had not reached the point where this substance could be properly tested and applied, the "sweet vitriol" of Lullus was actually ether, one of the most important of modern anesthetics.

Two centuries later, Paracelsus also produced ether in an

independent experiment. This Swiss physician, one of the giants of the late Middle Ages, was an avowed and outspoken enemy of dogma who taught his students at the University of Basel that, instead of blandly accepting the authorities of the past, they must test each truth and learn from their own experience. This brought charges of heresy against him and, in 1528, he had to flee Basel for his life.

A humanist with an insatiable curiosity, Paracelsus experimented continuously, seeking, among other things, some effective means of relieving pain. In one of his experiments he combined sulphuric acid with alcohol, distilled the mixture and tested the resulting "sweet vitriol" on chickens. Describing the results, he wrote: ". . . it has associated with it such a sweetness that it is taken even by chickens, and they fall asleep from it for a while but awaken later without harm. On this sulphur no other judgment should be passed than that in the diseases which need to be treated with anodyne, it quiets all suffering and relieves all pain . . ."

This same sweet vitriol, renamed "ether" in 1730 by the German, Frobenius, was also produced by the other brilliant German, Valarius Cordus, a younger contemporary of Paracelsus.

In his short span of twenty-nine years, Cordus left a memorable imprint on the emerging science of Europe. He helped set up a systematic science of botany, he helped speed the transition from alchemy to chemistry and he prepared one of the best pharmacopoeias of the period.

Although the ether discovered by Lullus and rediscovered by Paracelsus and Cordus was to wait another three hundred years before it was put to its proper pain-relieving use, a number of advances were made in the art of anesthesia during the late Middle Ages. Largely through the work of Paracelsus, atropine and mandrake were gradually abandoned in favor of opium, which he found more effective than other agents in relieving pain and anxiety, and these were used in operations until the anesthetic advent of ether in 1842.

While new pain relieving methods were being explored, old ones were returning into vogue. Pressure anesthesia, known from prehistoric times, was revived again. Ambroise Paré used this method as early as 1543.

About a year later, it was used by Realdo Colombo in Pisa. As described by the Spanish physician, Valverde, who was present, this was a strange performance. "The carotids," he wrote, "that is, the sleep-producing arteries, are so named because when they are pressed upon or closed up in any way we soon go to sleep. This experiment I saw performed by Realdo Colombo in 1544 in Pisa, on a young man in the presence of a number of gentlemen, with no less fear on their part than amusement on ours, for we gave them to understand that it was done by sorcery."

Pain relief by chilling, another method dating back to prehistoric times and used by Hippocrates, was reintroduced in 1646 by the Neapolitan physician and anatomist, Marco Aurelio Severino. The technique used was described by Thomas Bartholin of Denmark in his book, *The Medical Use of Snow*.

"Before employing cautery on wounds in various parts of the body, apply snow to dull the sensation . . . Severino had to apply the medication in narrow parallel lines; after a quarter of an hour the feeling would be deadened and the part could be cut out without pain."

Meanwhile, thanks to the upsurge of research in anatomy and physiology that came with the Renaissance, Harvey of England, in 1628, was able to make his brilliant demonstration of the almost total circulation of the blood, work which was finally completed in 1661 when Malpighi in Italy, aided by the microscope, discovered the capillaries. Once it was seen that the blood circulated through specific pathways which reached all parts of the body, a new concept of pain relief came into being. Instead of swallowing, inhaling or rubbing on a pain-relieving agent, would it not be possible to inject it into the blood and have it carried to all parts of the body?

Strangely, this proposal for intravenous anesthesia did not come from a physician but from the distinguished British astronomer and architect, Sir Christopher Wren, who is most famous for having designed St. Paul's Cathedral in London.

A methodical study of this technique was made by Johannes Sigmund Elsholtz, physician to the Elector of Brandenburg, who used intravenous injections of opium solutions. Because too little was yet known about human physiology and because the drug was difficult to control, there were some unfavorable results. After debate by the physicians of the seventeenth century, the method was temporarily put aside.

While the use of pain-relieving drugs underwent some improvement during the late Middle Ages and the Renaissance, major advances were made in anatomy and physiology. Actually, it was the great artistic surge of the Renaissance that made this possible. To paint the human body it was clearly necessary to know how it was formed, the placement of human bones and muscles, the mechanisms of tension and relaxation.

Leonardo da Vinci, unique among artists as among men, had the courage to perform a massive series of dissections upon human cadavers and make careful records of his observations. In the course of his monumental work, he dissected the cranial nerve and made casts of various portions of the brain. He found that sensation was carried by the nerves which he traced through the spinal cord. These nerves, he concluded, came together in a distinct portion of the brain. Without quite recognizing what it was, Leonardo also demonstrated the reflex arc which provides a protective reaction to pain before it is even perceived.

Leonardo's pioneering work in anatomy was ignored for a while, but swift, if troublesome, recognition was given the massive contributions of Vesalius, who later came to be known as the father of modern anatomy.

He, like Leonardo, performed a great number of dissections and, in the course of his work, continued mapping the nervous system and charting the various portions of the brain.

Even amid the great creative outpouring of the Renaissance, tradition and dogma buttressed the powerful fortress of ignorance. Vesalius was driven from Padua by colleagues who refused to tolerate his temerity in challenging the authority of Galen. Hounded by charges of heresy, he died in desperate circumstances on the Aegean island of Zante where he had been shipwrecked on his return from an expiatory pilgrimage to the Holy Land.

In France, where the use of herbal remedies to produce insensibility to pain was forbidden under heavy penalty during the seventeenth century, Nicholas Bailly, a barber surgeon of Troyes, was arrested for administering a narcotic to a patient before an operation and convicted of witchcraft.

Bailly's violation of authority was even condemned by a renowned colleague, the surgeon Guy Patin of the University of Paris, who protested to the medical faculty of Troyes: "If Bailly really uses narcotics in this way, you had better take him to task. See to it that these practices are not allowed, and do not let him go unpunished."

And in Scotland, as the seventeenth century was about to dawn, a lady of rank named Eufame MacLayne had her twin infants taken from her and was forcibly hauled up Edinburgh's Castle Hill. There she was chained to a stake and reduced to ashes. The charge against her clearly showed that she had employed a midwife named Agnes Sampson to provide her with "a certain medicine for the relief of pain in childbirth contrary to Divine law and in contempt of the Crown."

The paralyzing grip of dogma also reached into the New World, eradicating fact in defense of faith. It had been noted by the Spaniards that the Indians of Peru were able to relieve pain through use of the coca leaf, the source of cocaine. These reports were investigated by two Jesuits, Joseph Acosta and Antonio Julian, who found the coca leaf to be a truly effective agent in overcoming the sensation of pain. They documented their observations and sent them to the Church.

But the ingrained attitude of the religious authorities was

not to be shaken. In 1567, bishops from all over South America gathered at the Second Council of Lima and condemned the use of the coca leaf as false and contrary to religious dogma. Two years later, Philip II of Spain reinforced this with a Royal decree: "The notions entertained by the natives regarding it (coca leaf's pain-relieving properties) are an illusion of the devil."

Part IV

The Awakening Surge

Chapter 9

ON THE FRINGES OF SCIENCE:
HOAXES AND HEALERS

Pain hurts the same whether we explain it in magical or in scientific terms. And, at times, the magical healer can alleviate pain as effectively as the physician. Both may use opium; the witch doctor as part of a magical rite, the rational doctor as a drug able to deaden sensation. In either case the treatment is effective and the pain is assuaged.

The witch doctor, using opium as part of a traditional healing ceremony, may not realize that the drug would be effective without his incantations. The rational healer, for his part, might not appreciate the extent to which his concern and interest in treating the patient might, like the witch doctor's incantations, help ease the pain even without the effect of the opium. Sometimes the boundary between so-called magic and science is quite indistinct and may be more a matter of definition than of fact.

Yet there are clear differences between the two. Magic works because it works. If it fails, it is not the magic that is held at fault, but the client, the magician or some other force. Magic does not demand an explanation of itself. Science does. Science strives to be measurable, predictable, reproducible. Where magic accepts that opium plus incantation relieves pain and lets it go at that, science will test each separately to see if it alone can do the task. Then it will seek to determine why opium or incantation eases pain, how this is achieved, how the action can be controlled and finally, what this teaches us about the mechanisms by which the cure takes place. This not only helps us understand the drugs and techniques that ease pain but makes it possible to improve on them and even to develop entirely new approaches to the problem. This, if anything, is the great advantage of science over magic. Magic may work in certain areas but, because it demands only faith and does not constantly question itself, it remains relatively static. Science, constantly questioning and making new demands upon itself, is as viable as man himself.

The subtle and not-so-subtle distinctions between magic and science took on particular significance as Europe, still dragging some of the muck of medieval superstition, exploded into the period of rapid growth that led from the Renaissance toward the Industrial Revolution. Feudalism began to crumble before the pressures and demands of a developing society and an emerging middle class. New manufacturing techniques brought a need for better tools and machinery, larger supplies of raw materials, cheap and dependable power sources, more efficient transportation and communication. These needs prodded science into increased effort. The need for efficient navigation spurred the science of astronomy. The needs for better machines, dependable power sources, more useful metals, dyestuffs and so on stimulated chemistry, physics and mathematics.

This scientific development in other fields was bound to provide anatomy, physiology and the whole area of biology with new knowledge, tools and techniques. The all-important microscope was a case in point, as was the chemical process of oxidation which led to the understanding of respiration and other basic mechanisms of life.

Already, in the eighteenth century man's growing knowledge and technology were finally approaching the point where they would help him to learn the nature and mechanisms of pain and its transmission. He would no longer have to worry whether an herb was potent enough to relief pain, or so potent that it might kill. Instead, he would be able to determine the active pain-relieving agent in the herb, then extract and purify it so that it would have a predictable and reproducible action. But none of this had yet happened. Instead, man stood confused on the threshold to the future, as he had in Roman times.

Because of a gradually increasing recognition that sensation was transmitted by nerves, pressure anesthesia became somewhat refined in the eighteenth century. This time, instead of merely pressing the carotid arteries and producing unconsciousness by reducing the blood flow to the brain, a regional anesthesia was used, pressing nerves in the area to be operated upon. This had already been tried by Ambroise Paré in France, as well as by the seventeenth century Spanish surgeon, Valverde. In 1784, an advanced version was introduced by James Moore, an Englishman, who designed an apparatus that was said to be able to produce insensibility in various nerves within half an hour. A similar system was used with some success by the renowned British surgeon and biologist, John Hunter, in cases of amputation below the knee.

The Moore technique of nerve-compression anesthesia was evaluated by the British surgeon Benjamin Bell in his *System of Surgery*, which became a standard text in the eighteenth century. He felt that the method could only be perfected if a way were found to compress nerves without affecting the flow of blood. In his book, he also provided a useful summary of the existing methods of anesthesia. "The pain produced by operation may be lessened in different ways. By diminishing the sensibility of the system; and by compressing the nerves that supply the parts upon which the operation is to be performed . . . As opiates are apt to induce sickness and vomiting, I seldom venture on giving them before an operation, unless the patient has previously been in the habit of using them . . ."

There was much rough and ready surgery during this period, especially in view of Europe's competitive colonial expansion and its resulting welter of wars. On the battlefields and on the high seas, where medical facilities were rarely equal to the needs, rum, gin and whiskey were widely used anesthetics. Nor, lacking other means, was a sleep-producing blow on the head to be ignored. In any case, whatever the anesthesia, or even if none were used, many surgeons came to depend upon the sheer speed of their surgery. Dr. Langenbeck, Surgeon General of the Army of Hanover during the time of Napoleon, was reputedly able to amputate an arm at the shoulder in about the time required to take a pinch of snuff.

Because science, like mysticism, offers a key to the seemingly inexplicable, they are sometimes confused, especially where science is not yet supported by sufficient information.

The use of the will to ease pain must have seemed to verge on the miraculous to those who could not possibly know that we can condition our reactions and responses to a painful stimulus.

Something like this had been demonstrated by the seventeenth century French mathematician, Blaise Pascal. Suffering intense pain from a facial neuralgia, he found himself unable to sleep. Tossing in his agony, he remembered that Seneca, the stoic philosopher of Rome, had once commented: "The more the attention is fixed on the cause which produces pain, the more its intensity is increased; the more a man stands away from it, the more relief he gets."

In desperation, Pascal decided to test this and began to concentrate on a problem in geometry that had puzzled scholars for many years. In the course of his intense preoccupation he forgot his pain and solved the problem in one night.

Later, when he was asked to what use he would put his mathematical discovery, he replied: "None. But it was a good cure for a bad night."

Like Pascal, people who suffered pain wanted quick and effective relief. Most of them could not distinguish between science and non-science and they did not especially care. Nor could they wait for science to begin to achieve its promise, close as this might be. The intensely charged and socially volatile atmosphere of the eighteenth century was ripe for an increasing number of charlatans who mixed mysticism with pseudoscience, sex with salvation. The most notorious of these was the Sicilian imposter, Giuseppe Balsamo, who called himself Count Cagliostro. The most effective and the one who, inadvertently, made a distinct contribution on the borderland of science was the Austrian, Franz Anton Mesmer.

A tall, impressive, learned man who had graduated with honors from the Medical School of the University of Vienna in 1766, Mesmer took the idea of magnetism from physics, mixed it with the metaphysical concepts of astral and other heavenly influences, and combined these with the laying on of hands and other mystical concepts into a healing theory based on what he called "Animal Magnetism."

Witches were still being burned in Mesmer's day, the last being consigned to the flames in 1782. Another Austrian, Father Gassner, was achieving a vast number of "cures" by exorcising the devil out of the unfortunates who had been "bewitched" into illness and pain. Ranging himself against "superstition," Mesmer proclaimed himself a scientist who was, after all, using the newly discovered powers of magnetism.

He seemed to believe that the body, like the universe, contained a magnetic fluid. If this could be concentrated on the various aches and ailments, they would be cured. At the start, he actually used magnets in an attempt to harness these inner forces of animal magnetism. Later he decided that he was so filled with this force that he could transfer it to an object such as a stick, magnetizing it merely by passing his hands over it. Then he would point this wand at a group of patients; the animal magnetism would flow out and cure them of their pains and disabilities.

The Viennese medical fraternity denounced Mesmer as a quack and laughed him out of Austria. He thereupon went to Bavaria where the Elector, much impressed, appointed him a member of the Academy of Sciences. Then, in 1778, Mesmer came to Paris, with its decadent court hanging on the lip of disaster and with the mystical Marie Antoinette ready to become a devout follower.

The Duke of Bourbon and many other notable personages became followers of Mesmer. The Marquis de Lafayette even tried to introduce his theories into the United States. So many patients flocked to Mesmer for treatment that he could no longer deal with them singly and was compelled to introduce a form of group therapy.

By this time Mesmer had expanded his theories to include the belief that a patient must cooperate by "wanting" to get well. This helped him explain away failures. He also held that there had to be a rapport between patient and physician and that, in the course of the treatment, a crisis would be reached which had to be surmounted if a cure were to be achieved. In his strange way, he was putting down a foundation for some of the principles of modern psychiatry.

French medicine was highly skeptical of this bizarre form of competition. In 1784, a Royal medical commission investigated Mesmer's claims and discredited them. These findings were confirmed by the commission appointed by the French Academy of Science, which included the noted chemist Antoine Lavoisier and the distinguished American researcher in electricity, Benjamin Franklin.

Being exposed as a fraud should have ended Mesmerism. It did not. Bitterly disappointed by the attacks, Mesmer left France and retired on the wealth that his animal magnetism had drawn to him. But one of his devout disciples, the Marquis de Puységur, who was an amateur astrologer as well as a retired artillery officer, accidently stumbled onto a more serious extension of Mesmerism. According to some reports, the Marquis had paid Mesmer 400 louis d'or for his healing secrets.

Using Mesmer's principles, de Puységur "magnetized" a tree on his estate and people flocked to it from the surrounding countryside to be healed of their aches.

One day, an impressionable shepherd of fourteen, named

Victor Race, tied himself to the magnetized tree. The Marquis, who happened by at the time, stopped and stared at Victor intently, waving his hands before the youngster's face in an effort to add his own magnetism to that of the tree. Slowly the boy began to droop and passed into a trancelike sleep.

Surprised, the Marquis ordered the boy to untie himself. He obeyed, although he remained apparently asleep. The astonished Marquis then gave the hypnotized youngster other orders, all of which were carried out during the trance. Convinced that he had made a great advance beyond Mesmerism, de Puységur called his discovery "Artificial Somnambulism" and declared: "Hitherto, only drugs have been able to induce sleep. Through Mesmer's method of magnetism, I can now induce it."

A number of experiments were performed with this technique, which came to be called hypnotism. Unfortunately, its acceptance was hindered by association with charlatanism as well as the fact that it could not be adequately explained in terms of existing scientific knowledge. However, there were a few men with the courage to investigate its possibilities despite the risks that came with attempting something new and unpopular.

One of the most important applications seemed to be in the relief of pain. On April 12, 1829, the French surgeon, Jules Kloquet, first used hypnotism in surgery when he removed the breast of a woman after she had been placed in a trance.

In England, hypnotism was sponsored by one of the ablest physicians of the time, John Elliotson, Professor of Medicine at London University, who had introduced the use of the stethoscope to Great Britain.

What he did was considered unpardonable by his colleagues of the Royal Medical and Surgical Society of London. At his instigation, on November 22, 1842, a report was read to the Society by a Dr. Ward, detailing the successful amputation of a leg performed with the aid of hypnosis. The members of the group listened with growing indignation, refusing to credit the report just as they had refused to believe other reports of successful operations under hypnosis.

The quality of the scientific objections was probably best summed by a Dr. James Johnson who declared that he would not have believed the facts of the report even if he had been present at the operation and seen it himself. Another member of the Society, a Dr. Copland, declared that the paper should never have been read to them because, if it were true that the patient had felt no pain during the amputation, "the fact was unworthy of their consideration, because pain is a wise provision of nature, and patients ought to suffer pain while their surgeon is operating; they are all the better for it and recover better."

Because of his folly in attempting to introduce a new idea to his colleagues, Elliotson was forced to resign his post as senior physician at the London College Hospital. The whole affair led him to a profound and rather sad comment which, unfortunately, had a validity reaching far beyond its time and immediate target: "Our objects are of incalculable importance . . . the prevention of pain, in surgical operations . . . and possibly other advances. I feel no hostility to our opponents. They merely act the part of puppets . . . not knowing why they so act, and blindly obeying the general laws by which a supply of opponents to every truth and every improvement is always provided. The statistics of opposition to good things would show that their course obeys fixed laws; and they are to be pitied for being destined to the parts which they so eagerly perform."

Surgical hypnosis aroused far less hostility in the United States where a number of operations were performed with it. And, at a native hospital in India, James Esdaile, an English follower of Elliotson, used hypnosis as a means of anesthesia and, in a six-year period, performed several hundred painless operations, including amputations and other major surgery.

Had other events not been rushing to a climax, it is likely that hypnosis would have overcome the resistance to its use and won recognition as an important weapon against pain. Instead, under the impact of the new developments which ushered in the age of modern anesthesia, hypnotism was put aside and not revived again for pain relief until the mid-twentieth century.

At about the time Mesmer was stirring such great controversy in Vienna and Paris, the science of chemistry was at last reaching maturity. It was, among other things, on the verge of discovering the nature of air.

Air had puzzled man from earliest times. Some centuries before, Paracelsus had named air with the Greek word, *Chaos,* and out of this concept was derived the word "gas." The fact that air consisted of a number of different gases was simply beyond conception. Oxygen, as far as we know, was first extracted in 1678 by a Danish chemist named Ole Borch, who gets little credit for the discovery because he did not seem to know what it was.

A major breakthrough in the study of air came as the result of an advance in physics and mechanics, the development of an efficient pump that could produce a vacuum. This was achieved in the seventeenth century by a remarkable German, Otto von Guericke, who was also Mayor of Magdeburg.

Using the vacuum as a tool, the Irish chemist, Robert Boyle, and his assistant, Robert Hooke, began a study of the nature of air. They found that many phenomena that took place in air could not happen when air was absent. As they removed the air from a container in which a fire burned, the fire went out. And a living thing would die in a container without air. Obviously, there was something in the air that was necessary to both combustion and life.

Boyle decided that it was not the whole air, but a component he called "the little vital quintessence" that was the essential element. With the techniques and theory available to them, Boyle and Hooke had gone about as far as they could.

The next great advance leading to an understanding of respiration and the oxidative processes of life took place in

England in the 1770s. Joseph Priestley, a chemist who was also a dissenting Unitarian minister, heated the red oxide of mercury in a test tube and produced oxygen. As occasionally happens, this same discovery was made independently about the same time by Karl Scheele of Sweden.

In the course of his pioneering work on gases, Priestley also discovered nitrous oxide and helped lay the foundation for modern anesthesia. He even suggested that the inhalation of oxygen might be a useful treatment for certain diseases of the lungs. However, because of his independent religious views and his outspoken sympathies with the French Revolution, Priestley had to flee England after his house had been pillaged and burned. In 1794, he came to the United States, then a sanctuary for dissenters, and settled in Northumberland County, Pennsylvania, where he died in 1804.

Priestley's work with oxygen was rapidly expanded by the French chemist, Antoine Lavoisier and his brilliant wife. Using quantitative methods for the first time, they measured the amounts of oxygen entering and leaving the body and were thus able to determine the importance of this element in sustaining the processes of life. Equally valuable to science were the methods they introduced. These made it possible to study the effects and properties of many anesthetic and pain-relieving substances that came into use.

Just as Mesmer's animal magnetism rapidly gathered a cult-like following, a gas-inhalation vogue swiftly emerged from the suggestion that oxygen was essential to life and health. A number of legitimate physicians, along with an abundant sprinkling of quacks, took up the new "science of gases" as part of a fashionable and lucrative practice. Calling itself "pneumatic medicine," it attempted to treat a number of diseases such as scurvy, paralysis, cancer and even hysteria by making the patient inhale various gases which, in addition to oxygen, included nitrogen, carbon dioxide and others.

One gas, however, was avoided. This was nitrous oxide, which Priestley had discovered in 1771. This gas was shunned because an American physician named Lantham Mitchell had administered it to animals with disastrous results shortly after its discovery. Mitchell's conclusion that the gas was a deadly poison was accepted without reservation for more than twenty years. Then, a brilliant young Englishman of 17, named Humphrey Davy, decided to see whether the human species would react differently from smaller animals. He courageously inhaled the gas himself and, instead of dying, found himself enjoying the experience. He became pleasantly light-headed, his muscles relaxed, tensions seemed to leave him and his sense of hearing became sharper. In general, he felt so cheerful that he found it difficult to stop laughing.

Davy, who was later knighted, went to work as an assistant to Dr. Thomas Beddoes who had set up the Pneumatic Institute at Clifton, England, for the treatment of disease through gas inhalation. Although the Institute failed, the work done there by Sir Humphrey left a permanent imprint on scientific development as well as on the use of surgical anesthesia. He tested various gases then in use and sought to determine their actions. Using a device similar to that currently used to measure basal metabolism, he made a careful study of the effect of nitrous oxide on humans. He noted that inhalation of the gas caused a pronounced lack of oxygen and an increased expiration of carbon dioxide.

In 1800, Davy described the results of his extensive work in a book entitled: *Researches, Chemical and Philosophical; Chiefly Concerning Nitrous Oxide*. Here, for the first time, came suggestions for the use of this gas to relieve pain and produce anesthesia. He described how nitrous oxide was able to alleviate the pain of the gums resulting from an infected wisdom tooth. In another section of the book, Davy wrote: "as nitrous oxide in its extensive operation appears capable of destroying physical pain, it may probably be used to great advantage during surgical operations . . ."

With this observation regarding nitrous oxide, later known as "laughing gas," the age of modern anesthesia was finally heralded. But some time passed before the heralding trumpets were heeded.

In 1818, Sir Humphrey's equally brilliant student, Michael Faraday, noted that ether, then used for the inhalation treatment of some lung diseases, also had a soporific effect, something which Paracelsus had noted three centuries before and which had also gone unheeded.

Wrote Faraday in the *Quarterly Journal of Science and the Arts:* "When the vapor of ether mixed with common air is inhaled, it produces effects very similar to those occasioned by nitrous oxide . . ."

Although Davy and Faraday won great renown, it was as physicists rather than for the medical applications inherent in their work. Then, as always, the medical profession was jealous of its prerogatives and took a somewhat jaundiced view of any intrusions coming from outsiders. As it happened, even physicians or surgeons who disturbed the comfortable status quo with new ideas often found themselves in difficulty. This had been the case with Elliotson, who lost his post for advocating hypnosis; it came to be the case with Henry Hill Hickman.

A scholarly and serious young man, Hickman was admitted to membership of the Royal College of Surgeons in 1820, at the age of twenty. Fascinated by the possibilities of inhalation anesthesia, he started experimenting with carbon dioxide gas, using it on animals to see if it would actually ease the pain of surgery.

By 1824, Hickman had done enough work to show that certain gases, if inhaled, passed into the blood and could bring on an artificial sleep which would help abolish the pain of operation. He noted that it was essential to maintain a constant flow of blood in the patient and that the surgeon had to be prepared at all times to deal with the possibility of a circulatory collapse. All this he published in a pamphlet entitled *On Suspended Animation.*

Hickman's work was carefully done and well supported by experimental data. Unquestionably, he deserves credit for being one of the first modern investigators to show that gas inhalation could produce surgical anesthesia. But his work brought him only disappointment and frustration. There was little he could do to overcome the conservatism of the healing profession. The prejudices of the time were such that he found no surgeon willing to let him try this anesthesia on any of his patients. Despairing of British support, he asked the French Academy of Medicine to investigate his claims. Only Baron Larrey, the brilliant surgeon who had served with Napoleon, supported the youthful Englishman.

Resistance to change prevailed, but a change was certainly due.

Chapter 10

THE "DISCOVERY" OF SCIENTIFIC ANESTHESIA

Scientific anesthesia was born under a cloud of controversy, jealousy and greed. Bitter dispute raged over which individual deserved the credit and profit for having discovered it. The arguments were aired in the courts, in the streets and in legislatures. For a while it seemed that an important human achievement would be buried in the muck of scandal.

Anesthesia itself was never new, nor did any one individual invent or discover it. Pain relief began before the first man walked the earth and developed, empirically, through uncounted years of human experience. Many men contributed to the development of pain-relieving methods, but no one man invented them.

Nor did any single individual discover what we call scientific anesthesia. If one rather than another happened to be the first to use it, he was making an important contribution to the cumulative work of many men, in many fields, over many centuries. Lullus made ether in the thirteenth century. Was he the discoverer of scientific anesthesia? Or Paracelsus, who tried ether on chickens in the sixteenth century and suggested that it could be used to relieve the pain of surgery? Or Sir Humphrey Davy who wrote that nitrous oxide could be used as an anesthetic? Or Faraday? Or Hickman? Or the hundreds of others—Egyptians, Chinese, Indians, Greeks, Arabs, Jews, Italians, French, Germans, English, Americans and so on, who added to the accumulating store of knowledge that, inevitably, led to scientific anesthesia?

The question of who deserves credit for any discovery is too often distorted by personal emotion as well as considerations of nationality, race, religion and individual ego. Edison, certainly, could not have made an electric light without Galvani's prior work in electricity, von Guericke's vacuum pump, the early Phoenicians who are said to have discovered glass, and an uncounted number of other contributors to science and technology. The fact is that each discoverer or inventor, important as his own individual contribution might be, reaps from the crop of human knowledge and experience.

Everything necessary to scientific anesthesia was available for some time before its "discovery," waiting for someone to stumble across it and put it to use. And that, literally, is just about how it happened, through staggering and stumbling.

Davy had suggested the anesthetic use of nitrous oxide after he had tried it on himself and found that it had an intoxicating effect, making him feel lightheaded and lighthearted.

People disregarded Davy's anesthetic suggestion but took up the inhalation of nitrous oxide as a popular fad. It soon became fashionable to have "laughing gas" parties where people breathed nitrous oxide, or ether, which had a similar effect. It was a very amusing pastime. People inhaled the gas, became pleasantly intoxicated, staggered and stumbled about, talked foolishly, laughed loudly and lost some of their inhibitions.

The popularity of ether and "laughing gas" parties jumped the Atlantic and soon young people, especially students, had taken up the rage in the more populous areas of the Eastern seaboard of America. The whole business was so fascinating, especially because of its so-called "scientific" overtones, that patent-medicine pedlars and other itinerant showmen posing as "professors of chemistry" gave lectures and demonstrations which attracted the thrill-seekers and gullible in the small towns and villages of the countryside.

One such traveling showman was a tall young man of 18

with an incompleted preparatory school education. Decking himself out in a frock coat and a high hat, he proclaimed himself as "Dr. Coult of New York, London and Calcutta" and set out in 1832 to demonstrate the scientific wonders of "laughing gas."

With a home-made apparatus which he pushed about in a hand cart, he first toured the towns of Massachusetts, setting up in the public squares on market day and, after making a speech and demonstrating on himself, he would invite the spectators to inhale the gas. These spectacles so amused the audiences that Dr. Coult often collected as much as ten dollars when he passed the hat.

The young man, as it happened, was raising this money in order to be able to patent and produce a revolver he had developed. His name was really Samuel Colt of Hartford, Conn.

His laughing gas activities took him to many parts of the country. Once, as "Dr. Coult," on a Mississippi river boat that was threatened by an epidemic, he was forced to treat patients despite his pleas that he was not a physician.

A skilled showman, he became part owner of a penny museum in Cincinnati, where he put on a laughing gas show in order to help raise funds for Canadian patents on his Colt revolver. This time he decided to hire some Indians to inhale the gas, hoping that the novelty would attract a large crowd. He was right. The museum was jammed with people, many of whom came armed in the morbid expectation that the Indians would go on a scalping rampage.

What actually happened came as a shock to all. The Indians, probably having inhaled too much gas, promptly fell asleep. Colt, fearing the crowd would think itself cheated of its thrills and start a riot, quickly called a local blacksmith to the stage and gave him a whiff of gas. The befuddled smith then began to chase Colt around the stage, knocking over the Indians and waking them in the process. This saved the show.

Colt, bright young man that he was, did not realize that he had unwittingly anesthetized the Indians.

Fortunately, the strange effects of laughing gas parties and ether frolics were not entirely disregarded. Someone was finally bound to relate them to possible anesthesia. In 1839, a chemistry student named William E. Clarke, of Rochester, New York, started to entertain his friends with the effects of ether. He became so interested in the experiments that he continued them as a student at Berkshire Medical College. One day in January, 1842, he returned to Rochester where he decided to try ether on a young woman named Miss Robbie who was suffering a toothache. While under the influence of the ether, she had her tooth painlessly extracted by a Dr. Elijah Pope.

This, it would appear, is the first recorded use of ether anesthesia. It was reported by H. M. Lyman in his book, *Artificial Anesthesia and Anesthetics,* published in New York in 1881.

The first use of ether anesthesia in surgery was the subject of a monumental muddle at the start. When the original din and blather subsided and the facts were permitted to come into view, they pointed to Crawford W. Long. In the National Statuary Hall in Washington, D.C., Dr. Long's statue bears the inscription: "Discoverer of the use of sulphuric ether as an anesthetic in surgery, on March 30, 1842, at Jefferson, Jackson County, Georgia."

Long had come to Jefferson to set up his practice in 1841, shortly after his graduation from medical school in Philadelphia. Soon thereafter, a "laughing gas" showman intrigued the townspeople of Jefferson with a lecture on the strange effects of nitrous oxide. Anxious to try the gas for themselves, several people asked Dr. Long for a sample. As it happened, the young doctor did not have any on hand but he did have some ether, which, he assured them, would have about the same effect.

Some young men tried the ether in Long's office, became exhilarated, staggered about, laughed and behaved more or less as expected under the circumstances. But Long, more observant than most, noticed that as they staggered and stumbled about, bumping into furniture and bruising themselves, they seemed to feel no pain. Nor did he, himself, have any recollection of pain after joining the ether party and later finding bruises on his body. This set him to wondering about the possibilities of ether. If a small amount of it could mask the pain of a bruise, would a larger amount be able to prevent the more extreme pain of surgery?

Dr. Long answered this question on March 30, 1842. James M. Venable, a participant in the ether experiments, had some tumors on his neck which he had delayed having removed because of his fear of pain. Long suggested that the use of ether might permit a painless operation. Venable agreed to its use. That night Dr. Long poured some ether on a towel and held it over the patient's nostrils until he fell asleep. When Venable awoke, he was astounded to learn that one of his tumors was gone. He had felt absolutely no pain during its removal. The first operation under ether anesthesia was a success and the fee, incidentally, was two dollars.

During the next few years, Long used ether anesthesia in a number of operations, including some amputations. Although he did not publish his results, other physicians in the area knew about this work and followed it with considerable interest. The reason for Long's delay in publication was scientifically sound if personally unprofitable. He had been taught by his professors not to rush into print with anything that had not been fully verified by every possible means, so he had decided to wait until his results were beyond question. Consequently, a report on his work was not published until 1849, when it appeared in the *Transactions of the Georgia Medical and Surgical Association*. By then it was too late. Others were already fighting for the credit of having been the first to "discover" ether anesthesia.

Two years after Dr. Long's use of ether, Horace Wells, a dentist of Hartford, attended a nitrous oxide demonstration in New Haven. Like Long, he noted the curious fact that, after the subjects inhaled the gas, some of them fell and bumped themselves rather severely without apparently feeling pain. Intrigued by the possibilities of this fact, Wells tested the gas on himself and had a tooth extracted while under its influence. It proved to be a painless operation.

Wells was so pleased that he reported his findings to his close friend and partner, William T. G. Morton of Charlton, Massachusetts, a dentist who was also a medical student at Harvard Medical School. Wells continued to use nitrous oxide in dentistry until a patient died. Deeply depressed, he retired from practice and ended his own life.

Morton, who had been using nitrous oxide as a result of Wells' suggestion, began to look for a safer anesthetic. He discussed the matter with Dr. Charles Jackson whom he had met at Harvard, and was told about the pain-deadening properties of ether which Jackson had noted while attending several "ether frolics."

Seizing upon this information, Morton tried ether first on the family dog and then on himself. It seemed to work. The next step was to use it on a dental patient. He did this in September, 1846. The patient, Eben Frost, had a painfully infected tooth and, anxious about pain, asked that hypnotism be used. Morton assured him that ether would prove superior and, to the delight of both, this proved to be true.

There can be little doubt that Morton genuinely believed himself to be the first to use ether as an anesthetic. It is most unlikely that he knew of Clarke's use of it on a dental patient or of Long's use of it in surgery more than four years earlier. In any case, Morton's and Jackson's next step seemed motivated less by scientific modesty or the dedication of the healer than by the "me first and devil take the hindmost" attitude of the competitive anarchist. Adding several ingredients to ether in order to disguise it, they named the resulting product *Letheon* and applied for a patent which was later granted.

The enterprising Dr. Morton meanwhile prevailed upon the distinguished Dr. John Collins Warren to use *Letheon* on a surgical patient in Boston's Massachusetts General Hospital. The operation was performed on October 16, 1846, before an interested and distinguished audience. The patient slept throughout the operation and, even after he was revived, gave no indication of any pain. *Letheon* was adjudged to be an unqualified success.

Morton promptly published a paper and, supported by Dr. Warren and other highly reputable physicians and surgeons, was credited with the "discovery" of scientific anesthesia. Both he and Dr. Jackson were widely acclaimed throughout America and Europe; the French Academy of Science even awarded the Cross of the Legion of Honor to Dr. Jackson for his role in the discovery of ether anesthesia.

In order to reap a profit from the *Letheon* they had patented, Morton and Jackson planned to sell permits to physicians for fees of up to two hundred dollars. This caused a surge of indignation from the medical profession. Indignation became anger when doctors realized that they were actually dealing with ether, whose smell could not be disguised and which had been demonstrated at ether parties and by itinerant lecturers long before Morton could possibly have "invented" it.

It was not long before Morton and Jackson fell out, each claiming he deserved sole credit and profit for a discovery that had actually been made hundreds of years before. The disgraceful affair went into the courts and finally, in 1849, realizing that ether could not be protected by patent, Morton petitioned Congress to award him a substantial sum of money for his trouble and effort in providing mankind with this great boon. At this stage of the proceedings, Senator M. Dawson of Georgia came forward with evidence that neither Morton nor Jackson, but a physician named Crawford W. Long had been the first to use ether in surgery. Morton's petition was not granted.

Despite the facts revealed by continuing investigation, and even Jackson's admission in 1861 that the honor bestowed upon him by the French Academy rightfully belonged to Dr. Long, Morton continued to be hailed by many as the true "discoverer" of ether. This belief was buttressed by such eminent New Englanders as Oliver Wendell Holmes who, after the use of ether in Massachusetts General Hospital, coined the word "anesthetic" to describe the action of *Letheon,* and "anesthesia" for the state that it induced. Not until the end of the nineteenth century was the controversy finally resolved in Long's favor.

In this way, man's ancient labor for an effective, controllable anesthetic at last bore fruit in the New World.

Because of the distinguished men associated with the first use of ether in Massachusetts General Hospital, papers describing the event were quickly published in many important journals. News of the anesthetic "breakthrough" spread rapidly. Within two months after the Boston operation, ether was being used in England and, shortly thereafter, on the European continent.

The great importance of this new form of anesthesia lay in the fact that it was relatively easy to administer and control. Its effects were generally predictable, although accidents could and did occur, and it performed each of the functions required of a general anesthetic. It blocked the reflexive flinching that could be so dangerous during an operation, it entirely relaxed the body so there would be minimal resistance to the surgery, it eliminated the sensation of pain and, as an added boon, left no memory of the actual operation. The patient coming out of the anesthesia had no traumatic recollections to gouge scars upon his psyche.

The value of this advance was beyond question. But it was an empirical step forward, not one that had been made with forethought and foreknowledge. It had, in effect, been stumbled upon, tried and found useful. In this respect, the quality of the discovery—as distinguished from the importance of the object discovered—was little different from the Stone Age man's finding that the pain of a twisted ankle eased as he waded across a cold stream. Furthermore, Long, Morton and their contemporaries were hardly less ignorant than the Stone Age man about how their anesthesia was actually achieved.

The nature of ether's action, how and through which mechanisms it produced its effects, still remained to be discovered.

The dawning age of scientific pain relief was not universally hailed with hosannas. The inertia of tradition is even greater than that of matter, as even Sir Isaac Newton had cause to learn, and seems to increase as the square of its density.

Resistance to the new anesthetics developed swiftly. What followed is best exemplified by the experiences of a man who combined both the courage and brilliance to be able to meet the enemy on his own ground and there defeat him.

Dr. James Y. Simpson, who was later knighted, was professor of Obstetrics at the University of Glasgow, Scotland. He began to use ether to relieve the pain of childbirth almost as soon as he heard about its success in the United States. Upon administering it to several patients and finding the ether to have an unpleasant odor and irritating action, he looked about for a less troublesome anesthetic and decided upon chloroform, a then recent discovery by the illustrious German chemist, Justus von Leibig.

After successfully using chloroform in a number of especially difficult childbirths, eliminating what would have been considerable suffering and agony, Simpson published his results. Immediately he came under attack from all sides and from all levels.

This was no simple denunciation by the ignorant, which was to have been expected in any case. But the assault against Dr. Simpson came even from fellow physicians, from the clergy, from teachers, from the so-called enlightened and intelligent.

Newspapers, magazines and pamphlets joined to loose their arrows at him.

The resistance of many physicians to Dr. Simpson's use of chloroform in childbirth was due to the same causes that had prompted the attacks on Elliotson, hypnotism and other advances which, it was feared, might upset a comfortable status quo. The introduction of any element of possible change, they feared intuitively, could threaten their established procedures, practices and positions.

The substance of the charges leveled against Dr. Simpson arose out of the old religious and mystical attitudes which had plagued the development of mankind through the millennia. At the core of the attacks was the belief that the use of anesthesia in labor was an attempt to contravene the decrees of Providence, hence reprehensible and heretical.

An article published in the *Edinburgh Medical and Surgical Journal* in July, 1847, declared: "Pain during operations is, in the majority of cases, even desirable: its prevention or annihilation is, for the most part, hazardous to the patient. In the lying-in chamber, nothing is more true than this: pain is the mother's safety, its absence, her destruction. Yet there are those bold enough to administer the vapor of Ether, even at this critical juncture, forgetting it has been ordered that 'in sorrow shall she bring forth.'"

Even this serious medical journal, attempting to find justification for its defense of pain, took up a position behind the bulwark of theology.

A clergyman, denouncing Dr. Simpson from the pulpit, phrased the same argument somewhat differently. The use of chloroform was evil because it would "rob God of the deep, earnest cries which arise in time of trouble . . ."

Simpson neither retreated nor merely stood firm under the furious attack. A man who loved a hard fight in a good cause, he leaped to the counterattack. Extremely well versed in logic and theology, he examined the charges on religious as well as on scientific grounds. Then, in 1847, with accusations flying hot about him, he tore into them in a pamphlet entitled *Answer to the Religious Objections Advanced Against the Employment of Anesthetic Agents in Midwifery and Surgery.*

Detail by detail, Dr. Simpson demolished the theological arguments against anesthesia. He pointed out that the curses laid upon Adam and Eve in Genesis 3:16–19, ordaining that "In sorrow thou shalt bring forth children" and "Cursed is the ground for thy sake; in sorrow shalt thou eat of it . . . in the sweat of thy face shalt thou eat bread," were revoked in Deuteronomy 7:13 where it was declared that the Lord "will also bless the fruit of thy womb and the fruit of thy land . . ."

Simpson, a sound classical scholar, then went on to show that the original Hebrew word that was translated as "sorrow" actually meant "labor" and applied equally to the labor of childbirth and the labor of tilling the soil. Were the curse in Genesis to be accepted literally, as the defenders of pain were doing, then a man sinned each time he eased his labor by using an ox, a plow or even fertilizer to enrich the soil. Any labor-saving device was as much in contravention of the Lord's curse as pain-saving anesthetic.

Then he dealt with the belief, held by many doctors as well as clergymen, that it was wrong, sinful and immoral to use anesthesia because it produced a temporary insensibility, suppressing a divine spark of consciousness, merely for the purpose of "saving the patient from any bodily pain and agony."

The suppression of consciousness for the purpose of relieving pain did not at all violate God's will, Dr. Simpson pointed out. Instead, the reverse was true. According to Genesis 2:21, "And the Lord God caused a deep sleep to fall upon Adam; and he slept; and He took one of his ribs, and closed up the flesh instead thereof."

Lest there be any misinterpretation of the meaning of this particular verse, Dr. Simpson quoted John Calvin's *Commentary* which noted that in this first operation "Adam was sunk into a profound sleep, in order that he might feel no pain."

Dr. Simpson won his skirmish and the attacks against him subsided. But the fact that he had to take time from the important task of healing in order to answer such charges is an ironic commentary on the spotty progress of mankind's intellectual and emotional development.

At the very moment man was entering the great industrial revolution that was to transform the world and lead to today's scientific revolution, he was still beset with the superstition, ignorance and bigotry of his darkest past, albeit in modern garb.

Meanwhile, as Dr. Simpson was destroying the objections to the use of anesthesia, other pain-relieving agents were coming into use. The German pharmacologist, Friedrich Serturner, extracted morphine. This was the most active alkaloid of opium, the drug which Sir William Osler called "God's own medicine."

Atropine was isolated from belladonna in 1833 by the German, P. L. Geiger, providing an active pain-relieving agent similar to that hidden in the ancient mandrake and henbane. The coca-leaf, used by the Andean medicine men, yielded its active principle of cocaine. And, in 1853, C. G. Pravaz of France described the first hypodermic syringe.

New doors were opening along the corridors of knowledge, revealing vast new areas to be explored in man's conquest of pain.

Chapter 11

THE TIDE OF PAIN RETREATS

When nitrous oxide, ether and chloroform came into use, the Western world reacted as though anesthesia had been discovered for the first time. Even today, many of us still believe that anesthesia was introduced to the world in the nineteenth century by the Americans Long, Wells and Morton. Even Clarke, who preceded Long by several months, seems to have been forgotten.

Actually, anesthesia had been in use for thousands of years. It was easing the pain of surgery in Egypt, China and India long before America was first seen by Europeans and even before Europe had emerged from savagery. But, while the men of the eighteenth and nineteenth centuries may not have "discovered" anesthesia, they did give it a scientific dimension it never before had possessed. For the first time, the relief of pain was being brought under effective control.

A revolution in surgery began with the introduction of the new anesthetics. Until then, operations had to be brief and relatively uncomplicated because pain and shock were limiting factors. This gradually changed as surgeons attempted operations they could never dare risk before. These were not always successful and, in many cases, the effect of the anesthetic was not all that had been expected. Some patients even died as a consequence of the anesthesia itself. Obviously, much more remained to be learned. For anesthetics to be used safely and effectively, it was especially important to know how they acted, what adverse effects they had, how these effects could be minimized or eliminated.

Among the first three to begin such investigations were John Snow and Sir Benjamin W. Richardson in England and Claude Bernard in France. Snow, whose work on anesthesia and the actions of various pain-relieving drugs was published in 1858, had a rare distinction. He administered chloroform to Queen Victoria, winning Royal sanction for the use of anesthesia to ease the pangs of childbirth.

Bernard, who was born in 1813, the same year as Snow, was one of France's most gifted physiologists whose contributions enriched the whole structure of medicine. If the bright light Bernard shed was not so visible as it deserved to be, it was only because of the contemporary brilliance of Louis Pasteur. Yet the impact of Bernard's work upon medical science was no less important.

Bernard taught that the principles of biochemistry and physiology would have to be applied to win any understanding of the problems of life and death, health and disease. He was the first to propose that certain ductless glands produced internal secretions which were essential to the life processes. These we now know as hormones. He began an intensive study of the functions of the liver, pancreas and other organs and helped lay the groundwork for the investigation of digestive ferments, the enzymes.

In his investigation of anesthetic agents, Bernard was especially interested in determining how they worked and in what way they produced their effects. This, he felt, would help lead to an understanding of the mechanisms of pain and how these mechanisms might be blocked.

Recognizing that different drugs had different actions, Bernard sought to determine what these were. He was able to show that the drugs of the morphine group, the alkaloids derived from opium, eased pain in a different way from ether or chloroform. He even experimented with *curare*, the deadly arrow poison of the South American Indians, and showed that this acted by blocking the motor nerves, causing paralysis of vital muscles and organs. Today, curare is used in heart ailments and to produce complete muscular relaxation for long periods of time.

The fact that certain drugs could interfere with the nerves and prevent them from transmitting impulses was an extremely important finding because it revealed one of the major mechanisms of pain relief.

Like Snow and Bernard, Sir Benjamin W. Richardson investigated a great number of compounds for their anesthetic effect. However, because the techniques of making chemically pure drugs were still far from perfect, he found that the results were still not precisely predictable. Some of his most useful work was done in the field of local anesthesia. Recognizing that cold was able to reduce the sensation of pain, he began to experiment with different methods of chilling specific areas, rather than the whole body, without using ice packs or other cumbersome methods.

Since the process of evaporation withdraws heat from the environment and produces a chilling effect, Richardson tested a number of volatile liquids which evaporated very rapidly and thus produced cold. In 1867, he introduced the ether spray, an effective local anesthetic which was used for many years until replaced by ethyl chloride, which evaporates even more rapidly.

As all this work on anesthetic and other pain-relieving agents was gaining both attention and momentum, surgeons came to realize that an effective anesthetic had to do far more than just relieve the agony of an operation. In ancient times, before human physiology was clearly understood, pain relief had been considered enough. But as man gained more knowledge of himself, he began to realize that many complex body systems were involved in each life process and that these had to be taken into account whenever any method was used to relieve pain or to produce unconsciousness. Where this was not done, the patient was just as likely to die from the anesthetic as from the ailment.

A perfect general anesthetic, it came to be realized, had to do certain things and avoid doing others. In addition to eliminating pain, it had to produce complete unconsciousness as well as a deep depression of the central nervous system, so that pain-producing stimuli would not activate the reflex arcs. At the same time, the anesthetic had to have as little effect as possible on the reflexes which control respiration, circulation and other life-essential activities.

Furthermore, the anesthetic had to produce a very low state of muscle tone and complete relaxation of the abdominal walls. All these effects had to be achieved quickly, without setting up any undesired reactions and without interfering with the inhalation of adequate oxygen while the anesthetic was being administered. Finally, the effects of the anesthetic had to wear off quickly and completely, leaving no traces of its action and, most important, no memory of the operation itself.

No anesthetic has, as yet, met all of these specifications. Nor were all of these requirements known during the last century. The description of an ideal anesthetic has kept changing, and undoubtedly will keep changing, as we continue to learn more about the mechanisms and interactions of the life processes.

The problems of local anesthesia were far less complex and therefore simpler to approach. All that was needed was to depress or abolish sensation in a particular area such as a foot, leg, arm or jaw without causing adverse effects. This, it had already been shown, could be done by chilling, by pressing certain nerves and by the use of certain drugs. The medicine men of the Andean highlands had accomplished it by chewing coca leaf and dripping it into a wound.

Actually, it was this primitive drug that paved the way for modern local anesthesia in spite of some peculiar oversights and errors. In 1858, the active alkaloid principle of the coca, which had been known as "the divine plant of the Incas," was isolated in Germany by Albert Niemann and named *cocaine*. Neimann and Friedrich Woehler, in whose laboratory he worked, noted the fact that cocaine seemed to have a numbing effect on the tongue. Unfortunately, they did not recognize the possible significance of this. As a result, cocaine remained a medical curiosity for almost a quarter century.

Then in 1880, the British Medical Commission investigated the drug and reported that it had practically no medical value and was, at best, a rather poor substitute for caffeine. The next year, however, a contradictory report was published by Dr. Vasili K. Anrep of Russia, who indicated that cocaine might be useful in relieving pain in the eye.

It may be that Dr. Anrep's observation was brought to the attention of Dr. Carl Koller, perhaps not. In any case, Koller, an intensely modest man who somehow never received the credit due him for his work, was able to provide a clear demonstration of cocaine's value as a local anesthetic and help bring it into general use.

The demonstration of cocaine took place in 1884, only two years after Koller, a Czech, had graduated from the University of Vienna. Setting himself up to practice ophthalmology, he found an almost desperate need for an effective local anesthetic to be used in eye operations. Until that time, Richardson's ether spray was being used for local anesthesia but it had not proved satisfactory for work on the eyes. Koller began an intensive search for a new agent. His search seemed hopeless and he was on the verge of giving it up when his friend, Sigmund Freud, asked a favor of him. Freud wanted Koller to help him study the physiological effects of cocaine when taken internally. In the course of the tests, the ophthalmologist confirmed Dr. Anrep's observation that cocaine had a tendency to numb the tongue. Others had noted this and had dismissed it, but Koller could not forget it. Upon reflection, he decided that this might indeed be the anesthetic he was seeking. He began a number of experiments first on animals and then on humans, all of which proved cocaine to be effective as a local anesthetic.

The following year, after Koller had reported his findings to the Ophthalmological Society at Heidelberg, Dr. J. L. Corning of New York became the first to use cocaine as a spinal anesthetic, injecting a cocaine solution into the spine with the hypodermic syringe which had been developed by C. G. Pravaz in France and improved by Alexander Wood of Scotland. With this, a completely new technique of pain relief came into being.

The use of cocaine established, chemists immediately went to work to refine this derivative of the coca leaf still further, making more effective and less harmful extracts. This led the German chemist Alfred Einhorn to synthesize procaine, which is commonly known as "novocaine." The explosive growth of chemistry was bringing man to the point where he could actually create new substances, with predetermined characteristics that had never before existed in nature.

Meanwhile the revolution begun by nitrous oxide, ether and chloroform spread to many parts of the world. In Czarist Russia, it came to the attention of one of the outstanding men of the nineteenth century, Nicolai Ivanovitch Pirogoff, a scientist and humanitarian who helped bring light into a zone of darkness. Living at a time when it was illegal to teach the alphabet to peasants and working men, Pirogoff sponsored many "dangerous" advances, including greater freedom and opportunity for women. One of the eminent military surgeons of the era, he was so sickened by his battlefield experiences that he created the bitter epigram: "War is a traumatic epidemic."

A young prodigy, Pirogoff had passed the university entrance examinations at the age of fourteen with the aid of a forged birth certificate. This was necessary because the law had set sixteen as the minimal age for university admittance. In his first hospital assignment, he aroused such enmity by attempting to correct the horrible conditions he found there that the medical director accused him of insanity. Yet, by the very force of his intelligence and personality, he introduced a number of procedures which foreshadowed Lister's great development of antisepsis. He isolated infectious patients, shaved operative areas before surgery, advised against the common practice of exploring wounds with the fingers and used such antiseptics as alcohol, iodine and silver nitrate.

He was even involved in the introduction of women nurses on the battlefield during the Crimean War, at about the same time that Florence Nightingale appeared with her thirty-eight British nurses. The group of women organized by Pirogoff, in association with the Grand Duchess Helena Pavlovna, for the purpose of caring for the sick and wounded later became the Russian Red Cross.

In view of his humanitarianism and scientific originality, he welcomed the introduction of pain-relieving techniques and promptly looked for a new application. This search was spurred by a major problem of early ether and chloroform administration. These had to be inhaled through a towel or mask, which, for one thing, tended to interfere with the patient's breathing. But an even more serious objection arose from the fact that the administration of an inhalation anesthetic made it difficult if not impossible to perform operations on the mouth, nose and face in general.

Pirogoff studied the problem carefully and then published a historic paper on April 2, 1847, showing that "anesthesia could also be effective through the intestinal route." Instead of inhaling the ether, it could be introduced rectally through the technique now known as "rectal anesthesia."

After describing the method in detail, he outlined the advantages. ". . . it not only stops all sensations as easily and surely [as the inhalation method], but this end is obtained with less trouble for the patient and much faster it seems . . . the main advantage, of course, being that the respiratory system is not directly affected. No special apparatus is needed;

the action of the vapor is much less likely to be avoided [as in inhalation anesthesia where the patient can twist his head away]. Finally, the performing of many operations made difficult by the inspiration method, such as operations on the lips, mouth and face in general, are much facilitated."

For a while, rectal anesthesia did not gain much prominence, largely because ether was such an irritating substance. But when less irritating anesthetics were developed, such as the mixture of ether with carron oil and the later anesthetic, avertin, this method became very useful in many special areas of surgery.

As knowledge and techniques improved, it became increasingly apparent that special situations required special types of anesthetics. Consequently, as the demands became more refined and discriminating, newer and better anesthetic agents were developed along with more advanced methods of administering them. In the early part of this century, a "twilight sleep" using morphine and scopolamine became fashionable in obstetrics. This fell into disuse when it was found that it threatened the mother with post-partum hemorrhage and the infant with asphyxiation. Barbiturates were then introduced but, like a number of other agents, they ran into some serious objections.

Along with new drugs and techniques, there was a growing understanding of the nervous system, making it possible to relieve pain and relax the muscles in specific areas of the body. With this came caudal anesthesia, introduced in 1901 by M. A. Sicard of France, and developed through the first half of the twentieth century for obstetrics and more serious surgery. In this form of anesthesia, a nerve-blocking agent is introduced into the sacral canal at the lower part of the spine. More recent versions of this form of anesthesia make it possible to perform practically all abdominal operations and some chest operations without pain.

During this century, chemistry, biology, pharmacology, physics, physiology and other sciences have combined their information and skills to make the relief of pain practical and specific despite all of the complexities.

There are hundreds of different chemicals available which may be administered in a great variety of ways designed to meet the needs of many special situations. Anesthesiology has even evolved into an independent medical specialty, requiring the full attention of a physician soundly grounded in physiology.

While rapid developments in anesthesia were speeding the conquest of surgical pain, the far vaster realm of non-surgical pain was also coming under increasing control. The most widespread agonies by far are the less dramatic ones. Headache has probably been responsible for more sustained pain than all the world's amputations. Then, when we consider arthritis, inflammations, sprains, backaches, cancer and the uncounted other conditions that have beset man through the ages, we can see that the pain of surgery is a mere trickle alongside a torrent. Every human being, each day of his life, is subjected to some measure of pain.

Most of this is borne and passed away without too great stress. But where pain becomes intense, it is natural and normal to seek relief. Obviously it is not necessary to produce anesthetic insensitivity to cope with most headaches. The need is rather for some analgesic agent to raise the threshold at which we feel pain or diminish our reaction to the stimulus of pain.

The ancients produced analgesia in many ways; with infusions of willow bark, henbane, opium preparations and extracts from the snakeplant (*rawolfia serpentina*) to name only a few of hundreds of methods. Many of these, refined, purified or even synthesized, remain as modern analgesics.

The great upsurge in the development of pain-relieving and other drugs came, interestingly enough, out of the demands of the textile industry for better dyes. As a matter of fact, modern medications such as the sulfa drugs, oral anti-diabetes drugs and other so-called miracle drugs are offshoots of the chemical industry which produced aniline dyes from coal. As this industry developed in Germany, chemists learned to synthesize many things besides dyes from the products of coal tar. They reproduced products that existed in nature, they created new substances that had never before been known. Acetylsalicylic acid, which primitive medicine men had unknowingly extracted from willow bark to treat fever and aches of the joints, was synthesized from coal tar and, as aspirin, is used for the same purposes today.

The sweeping advances in chemistry that made possible the synthesis of utterly new drugs and pain-relieving agents was a direct reflection of the expanding science and technology that came with the Industrial Revolution. Prodding each other with new demands, they supplied one another with the ideas and materials to meet those demands. Out of this arose newer demands, newer ideas and newer materials. It became a continuing upward spiral which has led us into today's Scientific Revolution.

Inevitably, as part of this process, there had to come a growing understanding of the nervous system and the mechanisms of pain.

Part V

Modern Man Against Pain

Chapter 12

THE MECHANISMS OF PAIN

Through all the ages that man struggled against pain, until very recently he fought blindly. His main tools were time, patience and the techniques of trial and error. The successes he won were remarkable. He found opium, cocaine, India hemp, mandrake and a vast number of other substances that could produce analgesia or even deep anesthesia during which some of the most serious surgery could be performed.

All this success was achieved empirically. Man did it without knowing what pain was or how it was perceived. For the most part, all he knew was that a person felt pain under certain circumstances and that if he swallowed these substances or inhaled those fumes he would feel less pain or none at all.

For the greater part of his time on earth man did not know about the nervous system and the functions of the brain. Even until the early part of the nineteenth century, the possibility of understanding the nature of pain was confused by the tendency to relate the nervous system to consciousness and consciousness to the soul. And, where the soul was involved, science sometimes feared to tread. Clearly, many of the accretions of Western thought had to be unlearned and a number of attitudes modified before substantial progress could take place. Furthermore, a good deal of the ancient work, such as that of Herophilus and Erasistratus, had to be rediscovered.

Responding to the pressures of social, economic, technological and scientific change, the war against pain moved into increasingly rational channels.

The fact that certain nerves carry information and sensation to the brain, which had been noted by Erasistratus in the third century B.C., was recognized once more in 1811 by the Scottish anatomist Charles Bell who wrote that, "the nerves of sense, the nerves of motion, and the vital nerves, are distinct throughout their whole course, though they sometimes seem united in one bundle . . ."

One of the most valuable discoveries which led to an understanding of how nerves transmit their impulses came, as so often happens, by accident. In 1786, Luigi Galvani, a professor of medicine at the University of Bologna, hung some dead frogs on copper hooks outside a window. There happened to be a strong wind that day and it blew the frog's legs against an iron rail. Galvani, looking out of the window, was amazed to see the legs twitch every time they made contact with the iron. They reacted just as though they were being subjected to an electric current which made the muscles contract.

From this chance observation it became clear that muscles not only reacted to electricity but that electricity could be generated in animal tissue. The way now was opened for a scientific approach to animal electricity and the physiology of the nervous system.

This work was to be decisive in freeing the biological sciences from metaphysical captivity. It became apparent that many of the activities of the human body, previously believed under the supernatural influence of the soul, were actually subject to the natural laws of chemistry and physics. Neurology, the scientific study of the nerves, at last was able to take its place as a full member among the other life sciences.

After Galvani set the stage, another Italian, Alessandro Volta, and a number of other scientists turned their attention to the task of finding answers to the new questions introduced by electricity. What was its role in the life processes? How was it generated? Where did it act? What did it do?

Finally, in 1843, a German scientist with the French name of Emil Du Bois-Raymond was able to detect the existence of electric currents in the nerve tissue of frogs. Seven years later, Hermann von Helmholtz, who was also a German, succeeded in doing something that had been considered impossible—he measured the speed at which a nerve impulse travels.

The problem of pain came under attack from an increasing number of directions. Some of the most important pharmacological work was done by a most unusual Frenchman, François Magendie, during the first half of the nineteenth century. Opposing the belief that there was a single "vital force" that gave direction to life, he taught that the life processes had a physiological and biological basis which could be studied experimentally. He refused to accept any conclusions that had not been confirmed by experiment and was ready to carry his investigations into any scientific field in the belief that any data he found might be related to something else and help point the way to a new truth. Because of his readiness to probe for facts anywhere and everywhere, he dubbed himself a "ragpicker."

This vigorous collector of knowledge provided precious information regarding pain and its relief. Through a series of pharmacological studies into the sites of action of various drugs, Magendie was able to show where in the body particular drugs acted. He was also the first to show which nerve roots of the spinal cord affected motion and which nerve roots dealt with sensation.

Meanwhile, on another front against pain, scientists were attempting to map the complexities of the nervous system. The problems involved here were almost beyond imagination and, even with today's discriminating techniques, are still far from solved. Each nerve pathway and relay, it was found, carries a specific type of information. Nerves that carry sensation, for instance, handle one particular type of sensation and no other. The nerves of touch follow different pathways from those of pain. The nerves which order a particular muscle to relax are different from those that order it to contract.

Imagine a communications system in which each particular

type of information and each separate kind of response requires a distinct and independent channel! This is the complexity of the nervous system, normally functioning so efficiently within us, that the neuroanatomists had set out to chart.

A number of pathways were traced, including those of pain, as they traversed the main trunk of the spinal cord to the particular areas of the brain that processed the information they carried. While this work was being done, other scientists were framing experiments that asked a different set of questions. What were the biochemical processes which helped a nerve cell transmit its impulses and how did the cell receive the energy needed to do this work? The answers would help lead to a better understanding of an important mechanism of pain, as well as to several possible means of blocking it.

The coca leaf, for instance, which had been used in primitive times and which, as cocaine, became an effective local anesthetic, had been a mystery as far as its mode of action was concerned. Trial and error had shown it to be effective against pain, but how it did this was simply not known. The same was true of other anesthetics and analgesics. But once the chemistry of the nervous system began to be understood, it was possible to see how the coca leaf, cocaine, novocaine and a number of other pain-relieving substances worked.

They eased pain not by doing anything about the pain stimulus but by interfering with the chemistry of the nerves which carried the impulse. In this way they set up a block, actually a nerve block, that kept the message from getting through to the brain.

This is by no means the only method that can be used to interfere with the mechanisms and pathways of pain. There are a number of others which have come to be understood and even more, undoubtedly, that are still to be recognized. But in the early nineteenth century the first important breakthrough had just been achieved.

Other scientists came into the picture. Studies on how impulses were conducted through the nerves and spinal cord to the brain were refined and extended by such men as Keith Lucas of Cambridge, who was killed at the height of his career in the first World War. His work was carried on and extended by E. D. Adrian and G. R. Mines in England, as well as by Joseph Erlanger and Herbert S. Gasser in the United States.

Extremely important contributions to this knowledge were made by Sir C. S. Sherrington of Britain and Ivan Pavlov of Russia, whose memorable research into conditioned reflexes showed how reactions to pain may develop and how they can be modified and changed.

Then, with the work in England of T. R. Elliot and Sir H. H. Dale, the Austrian-born Otto Loewi, and other dedicated researchers, the chemical mechanisms of nervous transmission came into clearer view.

Much of this vital work dealt mainly with one part of the problem of pain, how it was stimulated and transmitted. At least as important was still another aspect of the total problem, what happened when the pain impulse reached the higher centers of the brain where it was recognized, interpreted and where a reaction was set into motion.

The complex task of mapping and localizing the sensory areas of the brain made considerable progress thanks to the investigation of Sir Henry Head in Great Britain and Max von Frey of Germany. And, within the last few decades, remarkable advances have taken place in tracing the brain's relays and switching operations that compare incoming impulses with stored memories of identical or similar experiences and, on this basis, set up the patterns of reaction to a particular event. This work, conducted by a growing legion of such exceptional men as Wilder Penfield of Canada, W. S. McCulloch and H. W. Magoun of the United States, P. K. Anokhin of Soviet Russia, and others still has far to go, but its implications are enormous since it deals with the most basic mechanisms of learning, thought and behavior.

After all the millennia of pain we can at last begin to see its nature. True, the total picture is still far from complete, but the major mechanisms are visible and some of the pathways can be traced almost in their entirety.

Pain begins with a particular type of stimulus to a special type of nerve ending. These are the pain receptors and they are unlike those of touch and temperature because they are naked nerve fibers without any specialized structures at the tip. There are pain receptors throughout most of the body. Millions of them lie in delicate loops just under the surface of the skin. Others are in the mucosa, in the body's interior, in the blood vessels and organs.

These nerve endings are the body's windows on pain. Without them we could be stabbed, cut, clubbed, burned or chewed and would feel no painful sensation whatsoever. Neither arthritis, angina nor a rupturing appendix would cause us any agony.

The receptors of pain are not uniformly distributed throughout the body. Unlike the receptors of touch, which are more plentiful at the hands, feet and other peripheral areas, the pain ends are more highly concentrated in the parts more sensitive to injury. The tip of the nose or the palm of the hand may have between forty and seventy of these so-called pain spots in each square centimeter of skin, but the groin or armpit will have some two hundred pain spots in an equal area. We are more sensitive to pain in the parts of the body having a higher concentration of pain receptors. What would feel like a light, painless tap on the sole of the foot, where there are relatively few pain receptors, would seem a painful blow if inflicted to the groin and would be absolutely agonizing in the eye. The logic of this is obvious. Without such a highly functional distribution of pain receptors, developed through ages of natural selection, the act of walking would be utter agony to our feet, while the delicate structure of our eyes would be far more vulnerable to destruction without their multiplicity of pain receptors.

The pain endings are not selective as are the other sense receptors. They will respond to almost any type of stimulus provided it is intense enough to cause or threaten injury. Gentle pressure on the palm of the hand will only stimulate the nerves of touch. But if the pressure increases to a point of danger, the pain receptors are aroused.

Each nerve end is the start of a chain of nerve cells that forms a particular pathway of pain. Very much like a telephone line, it carries messages from one station only and these messages go out on an individual wire. Continuing the telephone analogy, the individual pain "wires" from an adjacent area join into branches, branches join into trunks and they all enter the central nervous system through the nerve roots of the spine or the nerves of the head. The spinal cord actually serves as the main cable of the nervous system, carrying thousands upon thousands of separate and distinct nerve "wires," each one of which is a communications link between one particular part of the body and a corresponding part of the brain.

The pain receptors, like nerves of other senses, do not send out an impulse unless they receive a stimulus strong enough to excite them. The level of stimulation just strong enough to start this activity is known as the pain threshold. Here we come to one possible mechanism through which pain can be relieved. Any agent that can raise the threshold of the pain receptors will serve as an analgesic.

Oddly, the pain threshold is pretty much the same in all people under normal circumstances. Tests have shown that the supposedly stoical Indian and the high-strung neurotic who can barely endure the thought of pain need about the same amount of stimulus to start a pain impulse on its path. The difference between them becomes apparent once the impulse reaches the brain and is interpreted and "felt." The reaction to this message can vary widely between individuals and even differs in the same individual at different times, because the interpretation of a sensory message involves emotional and other highly personal factors.

In practical terms, we could probably sum this up by saying that while the pain threshold is generally similar in people, the reaction threshold is subject to wide variation. One man will barely notice a nudge in the side with an elbow, another man will react as though his rib had been caved in. In both cases the stimulus was the same and the intensity of the impulse reaching the brain was the same. The difference was in reaction threshold.

When a pain receptor is excited by a stimulus, a chemical reaction takes place in the nerve. The precise chemical changes that occur are not yet clear and are currently being studied. But it is known that these changes produce an impulse which is invariably accompanied by a minute but measurable discharge of electricity. The impulse in one cell acts as a trigger that sets off an impulse in the next cell and so on along the nerve pathway until the impulse reaches the brain. The energy for an impulse, which moves along a nerve pathway much as a spark moves along a fuse, comes from chemical activity within each nerve. And the speed at which the impulse travels, first measured by von Helmholtz, depends upon the thickness of the nerves and the kind and size of creature involved. It is slower in cold-blooded than in warm-blooded animals. In humans, the speed of a motor nerve impulse may be as high as one hundred and ten or more yards a second. Pain impulses move at a somewhat slower pace.

It may seem strange, but the impulse generated by a very weak stimulus has the same intensity as the impulse of a powerful stimulus. The impulse produced by a pinprick is the same as that of a saber slash. The difference is not in intensity but in the number of impulses. The message traveling along a nerve pathway does not flow as a steady signal but in bursts of impulses, the number depending on the strength of the stimulus. This may vary from ten impulses per second to a thousand. Thus, the pinprick may send out twenty impulses per second while the saber slash could reach the limit of a thousand. Here we can see a second possible area for the relief of pain. Any agent that can lower the metabolic activity in the nerve cells and so decrease the number of impulses per second will serve to ease pain or stop it.

According to sensitive measurements, one thousand impulses per second actually represents the limit carried by any nerve. This would imply that there is a cut-off point beyond which the real intensity of pain or other sensation cannot increase. The absolute limit of pain any of us can receive is the same. No normal person can, literally, "take" more pain than any other normal person. The apparent differences lie in individual reactions to the pain, the extent to which an individual may condition himself or be conditioned to endure.

As a pain impulse begins to move along its pathway it will, if it is a surface pain, pass through a special nerve structure known as a reflex arc. This arc acts as a sort of emergency relay station, permitting the pain impulse to pass on its way to the higher nervous centers while, at the same time, starting a nerve impulse going back to the area where the pain stimulus was produced. This returning impulse is motor rather than sensory and it carries instructions for action in response to the information that aroused it. Traveling along its own nerve pathway, this reflex impulse stimulates a muscle or set of muscles to flinch or take some other protective action against the cause of the pain. There are hundreds of thousands of such reflex arcs in our bodies and they act before the information of pain has reached our brains. However, as Pavlov has shown, we can condition ourselves to modify or even change our reflex responses.

In a sense, they may be compared to a fire sprinkler system which is set off automatically when the heat rises above a designated level; and only then, after it has been set off, does an alarm sound at the fire station.

After passing through the reflex arc, the pain impulse continues along its pathway into the main trunk of the spinal cord or through one of the cranial nerves. All these paths lead into the brainstem where the impulse passes through a nerve network known as the reticular formation. Here the pain begins to enter the consciousness as the impulse triggers arousal or awareness signals of something wrong. The actual feeling of pain does not come until the impulse passes into the great receiving center of the brain, a sort of main switchboard known as the thalamus. Now the source of the pain impulse is localized, the tip of the index finger for instance, and the impulse is then switched to the appropriate part of the cerebral cortex for interpretation, processing and reaction. Here the pain reaches its full meaning to us. Not only do we become fully aware of it and its location, but we compare it with stored memories of other sensations and reactions, draw forth emotional responses, and bring together all the data that will let us know how intense the pain seems to us and set the patterns of interpretation and reaction. Here our total experience and personality come into play, our past encounters with pain, our associations, attitudes, moods, emotional status, anxiety, judgments and whatever else helps make us what we are at any given moment. It is at this point that the stoic will decide to disregard the pain while the highly sensitive individual will scream in anguish. And it is here that we take the conscious action, if any, to stop the pain or to remove its cause.

At this level, too, pain can be blocked out by using drugs or other anesthetic agents to depress the consciousness so that incoming pain impulses are simply not processed or even recognized.

The mechanisms of interior pain, as they are still incompletely known, are somewhat different from those of the body surface. The receptors of deep pain do not seem to be stimulated by piercing or cutting but are activated by pressure, chemical irritation, inflammation, stretching and other distortion. Nor does interior pain activate any protective reflexes.

The solid organs of the body seem to be completely insensitive to pain stimuli. But the hollow and tubular organs, the blood vessels, viscera and certain supporting tissues contain pain receptors that send their impulses through the nervous system.

Failure of the blood to remove chemical wastes from muscles and joints will produce inflammation and excite the pain receptors. The distention of an inflamed appendix or of indigestion will activate pain impulses. And a circulatory inadequacy may distort certain blood vessels and bring on the pain of angina pectoris.

Pain impulses from the interior enter the main trunk of the spinal cord leading to the brain. At that stage they can be depressed, slowed or stopped by nerve blocking anesthetics injected into appropriate parts of the spine.

When the interior pain impulse enters the brain, it follows the same general pathways and processing as surface impulses. But there are some differences. Interior pain seems more diffuse and is more difficult to localize than exterior pain. Even without looking, we can know precisely which part of which finger has been hurt. But we cannot say with any certainty whether an abdominal pain is centered in the stomach, intestine, duodenum or the gallbladder.

There is another strange phenomenon of pain that should be recognized. This is the matter of referred pain. We may feel pain coming from one part of the body when, actually, the pain stimulus is being applied somewhere else. This may happen in a number of ways.

If a particular nerve pathway leading from the big toe of the left foot is excited by pressure or chemical activity at some point, say as it enters the spine, an impulse will be started along that pathway. When it reaches the brain, this impulse will be identified as coming from the big toe. Pain will then be felt in the big toe although the pain-causing stimulus is actually in the spine.

Referred pain is also felt in "ghost" limbs for some time *after* an amputation. This results from the continuing activity of the remaining nerve pathways which had led into the amputated limb. And a considerable number of headaches are actually the results of referred pain from some other part of the body. Digestive upsets, for instance, often produce headache.

Pain, as we now are well aware, can also be caused by mechanisms in which the emotions are involved. Emotional activity interacts with the body's biochemistry both as a cause and as an effect. Certain changes in hormonal balance, fluid balance or in the over- or underproduction of body chemicals will produce certain changes of mood. And, working the other way, certain emotional stimuli will bring about a number of chemical reactions. Anxiety can cause a set of changes which will increase or decrease the pressure of body fluids. This can excite the pain receptors in the area involved and produce a headache, stiff neck or a pain in some other part of the body.

Such pain, instigated by factors that we call emotional, usually follows the same pathways as so-called somatic pain and is, in fact, produced by the same physiological activity and uses the same biochemical and neural mechanisms. Today's deeper knowledge of the integrated totality of the life processes leads us farther and farther away from the mystical-religious concepts that divided the living organism into two distinct parts, the body and soul, the *soma* and the *psyche,* the physical and emotional.

Instead, we are constantly being brought closer to the understanding of life's unity—that what we called physical and emotional are part of the same totality and abide by similar laws. Anger, love and thought, no less than the circulatory, respiratory or digestive processes, all take place within the biochemical and mechanical structures of the body, utilize oxygen to help supply their energy needs and produce carbon dioxide and other wastes as their metabolic byproducts. And pain, too, utilizes similar biochemical and bioelectrical mechanisms, whether stimulated by the pricking of an anxiety or the pricking of a thorn.

Chapter 13

THE INTERPRETATIONS OF PAIN

"Feeling" hurt is by no means the simple thing that it sounds. By the time a pain impulse enters the level of our consciousness and becomes felt, it has undergone a processing so intricate that we can only guess at many of its complexities.

Localization of pain, comparison, evaluation of intensity, interpretation and reaction are all involved. These, in turn, are influenced by past experience, present condition and the interaction of many other factors of which we are but dimly aware. We may stub a toe during a depressed state and barely feel it. Another time, also during a depressed state, a similarly stubbed toe may produce great agony. Why should the same emotional state make us feel pain differently at different times?

Fatigue also has an unpredictable influence. Sometimes we may be too tired to feel anything. Another time, equally tired, the slightest pain becomes magnified beyond endurance.

Clearly, while the mechanisms of pain are excited more or less equally by an equal stimulus, the manner in which we interpret and react to pain—"feel" it—is modified by many constantly changing relationships. Science has barely begun to identify and measure what all of these may be.

The biochemical and bioelectrical changes involved in the various emotional, fatigue and health states are almost beyond the range of calculation. Determining the number of possible combinations of the varying states of being, each with a different set of reactions, would probably tax the most sophisticated computer to the limit of its capabilities, or beyond. Yet each one of these must certainly affect and be affected by the biochemical and bioelectrical mechanisms involved in the way we feel, interpret and respond to pain.

The brain, wherein our responses and feelings of pain are determined, is subjected to an almost infinite number of influences. Scientists exploring the mysteries of the central nervous system sometimes visualize the brain as a complex living data-processing computer with self-programming capabilities. Like the purely electronic computer, it has inputs, outputs, memory banks, an incredible web of connecting circuits, delicate switching mechanisms and relays. In many practical ways, the analogy is very close. But where a giant computer may have several million electronic elements, the human brain has an estimated one thousand billion neural elements and its switching time, the time required to speed impulses from one group of elements to another, is estimated in ten-thousandths of a second.

In so complex a mechanism, with so many parts and connections, the slightest chemical changes or pressure variations could slow a switching operation a fraction of a second, momentarily inactivate a needed neuron, send too strong or too weak an impulse into a nerve circuit or stimulate the wrong memory cell. The possibilities are endless and they account for numberless variations, most of which, because we are as yet unable to trace their mechanisms, are unpredictable.

All this may seem to verge on science fiction but its reality has already been demonstrated experimentally in a number of ways.

In an unusual piece of research performed in 1958, Wilder Penfield of McGill University in Montreal sent mild electrical impulses into the brains of a group of people. These impulses were directed into the specific areas where memories are stored. Under the stimulation of the current, the brain cells released their memory data into the centers of consciousness, not as memories of long past or recent events, but as experiences which the people actually relived in their consciousness. This was not simply a matter of the people remembering the sights and sounds of a previous experience, but of their apparently seeing those sights and hearing the sounds as though the actual event were then occurring. It was in no way an hallucination that they sensed.

This may be an extreme example of how unusual stimulation can produce changes in the brain mechanisms involved in our thoughts, interpretations and reactions. Yet it does show that such phenomena can be produced by gross stimuli from outside, and must certainly indicate that similar events can and do occur as a result of the far more numerous and subtle changes within the organism.

Electrical stimulation of particular brain centers has produced violent anger, joy, depression and other emotions and moods. Some very recent research by Dr. James Olds of the University of Michigan has shown that there is an area in the brain which, if stimulated, can produce feelings of intense pleasure. Animals with electrical probes stimulating these "pleasure centers" are willing to suffer otherwise unbearable pain or even die of starvation rather than surrender this pleasure stimulus.

Experiments with pain have shown that people can feel pain even where no actual pain stimulus exists. An electric impulse sent into the spine at a point where it will irritate the nerves of a pain pathway coming from the ball of the foot, for instance, will make us feel a sharp pain in the foot, a very real pain no different from one caused by stepping on a tack. And we may feel, interpret and react to it just as if we *had* stepped on a tack.

Localized centers of the brain that process pain impulses from particular parts of the body can also be stimulated electrically so that we will actually "feel" pain in those parts— the arm, back, nose, lip, tooth, neck and so on. In all of these cases, what happens is similar to a short circuit in a switch which turns on a specific pain response mechanism.

All these factors can give us only the sketchiest idea of what might be involved in the presumably simple matter of "feeling" pain. And when two people have sharply different reactions to the same pain stimulus there might be a great number of possible reasons. Actually, the nerves which transmit pain may be implicated. Fatigue, or other conditions, might lower their metabolic activity so that their normal ability to send impulses is temporarily impaired. A stimulus that ordinarily brings a response of ninety impulses per second might in such a case produce only half of that number of impulses per second. The intensity of the pain is thereby cut in half, although the stimulus is the same.

Differences in the way we "feel" pain might also depend on the way the cerebral cortex is able to control the thalamus. Many scientists agree that the cortex is the highest brain center, the part involved in thought, intelligence and the more deliberate activity. The thalamus, on the other hand, lying deep within the brain, is a more primitive center that emerged in an earlier stage of evolution and around which the more complicated brain structures have since developed.

In addition to being the great receiving and distributing center for incoming impulses, the thalamus is a seat of emotional display and reflex activity. Millions of years ago, before intelligence developed, the thalamus might have served as a brain that could spur a creature to swift reaction triggered by intense emotions of fear, rage or hate. Today, uncontrolled, it could make us wild with fury, ungovernable with passion or hysterical with pain.

With the cerebral cortex exercising control over the thalamus, we become capable of considered behavior and reasonable reactions to various situations, including those of pain. If we have been sick or under some great stress, the control over the thalamus may lessen and our responses to pain and other stimuli become exaggerated.

In such a state, with the more primitive levels of the consciousness taking over, imagination can quickly produce panic.

Wild warnings could flash in our brain: "They are going to hurt me again. I cannot stand pain. This is torture! They mustn't touch me!"

Failure to respond to pain can be just as abnormal as an overreaction. Depressed responses can be conditioned, or they may result from physical or emotional disturbances. There have been cases of people whose pain mechanisms simply stopped working and they could be jabbed with needles or spattered by molten metal without feeling a thing.

The American Indians, according to some researchers, were conditioned almost from birth not to respond to pain. This does not mean they were impervious to pain, they certainly did feel it. But they were better able than many others to control their reactions.

Professional boxers tested in New York also seemed less reactive to pain than average. This, too, was probably due to conditioning as well as the fact that such a violent calling would be more likely to attract underreactive individuals.

The so-called emotional components of the pain response can have a powerful influence on what we feel. Dr. Henry K. Beecher of Harvard Medical School reported in 1962 that three-fourths of the men who suffered great wounds at the Anzio landings in World War II did not feel sufficient pain to want anything done about them. Apparently, the fact that these wounds meant release from the greater horror of the war affected their interpretation of the pain, lessening it.

Hysteria, too, can depress the consciousness of pain. In 1920, Dr. Theodore Diller of the United States wrote in *The Journal of Abnormal Psychology* that during the First World War, some soldiers under severe fire felt a peculiar numbness in various parts of their bodies. When tests were performed on these men it was found that they had lost all sense of feeling in those areas.

Under the stimulus of athletic competition, anger, fear, sexual excitement or any extreme situation that involves a burst of thalamic activity, the processing of pain impulses may be sidetracked and pain, consequently, not felt. Intense mental concentration can also depress one's awareness of pain by focusing the activities of the cerebral cortex into another area. This, presumably, is what happened when the French mathematician Blaise Pascal was able to escape the intense pain of his ailment by solving a problem in geometry.

Mental illness, in which the brain's ability to process data is impaired, can also have a profound effect on the ability to interpret and respond to pain. On March 19, 1958, Dr. W. E. Marchand and a group of associates reported in the *New England Journal of Medicine* on a study made of 79 psychotic patients who were suffering from acute perforated ulcers, acute appendicitis or fracture of the femur. Those three conditions normally are intensely painful. Yet, more than one-third of the patients felt no pain whatsoever. In their case, it would seem, the ability to recognize and respond to pain had been lost.

The great range of variation in pain response, determined as it is by vaguely understood interactions in the various structures of the brain, is said to be "subjective" in nature. What this really means is that we know too little about the processes involved and still lack the means to make any reasonably accurate observations, measurements and predictions. Once any phenomenon becomes scientifically predictable, it quickly seems to lose its semi-mystical aura of subjectivity.

Something like that happened in 1952 to the questions of pain intensity and the threshold of pain sensation. That year, at the Cornell Medical Center in New York, Drs. J. D. Hardy, H. G. Wolff and H. Goodell developed a sensitive test for measuring the threshold of pain. Using an electric projection lamp, they would focus its light on a blackened spot of the subject's forehead. This produced the sensation of warmth. They would then increase the current in the lamp until the warmth became a jab of pain. The heat that produced this threshold sensation of pain was then measured in millicalories (thousandths of a calorie) per second on a square centimeter of skin.

After testing a number of people over a period of time, the Cornell scientists found that the threshold value of pain is pretty much the same in all people. Boxer and ballerina alike start to sense pain somewhere between 210 and 230 millicalories when the light is applied to the forehead. This threshold varies at different parts of the body. The finger and toe threshold is about 300 millicalories while the eye begins to feel pain at 25 millicalories.

With this device it has become possible not only to test pain thresholds as such, but to study the effects of emotion, fatigue and various drugs on the ability to perceive pain. Men and women show the same threshold of sensitivity. Race, nationality or occupation seem to have no influence. Age does cause a difference and sensitivity decreases with the years. Emotions do not appear to change the threshold much; fatigue does, but in ways that cannot be predicted. Certain analgesic drugs such as morphine, codeine and others seem able to raise the threshold of pain. The threshold in one part of the body can be raised by discomfort in another part. A person with a toothache will be less likely to feel the pain of a stubbed toe. And the irritation of the skin by a liniment may reduce the pain of an aching muscle.

In addition to measuring the thresholds of pain and finding them generally uniform in all people, Dr. Hardy and his associates also adopted a scale that measured the whole range of pain. Earlier work had shown that from the threshold to the absolute maximum of pain, there were twenty-one perceptible increases of intensity. Each two of these steps became a unit of pain intensity known as a "dol," after *dolor,* the Latin word for anguish. From the threshold on, the entire intensity range of pain covers 10.5 dols. It is here, in the number of dols which a person is able to bear, that the response to pain may vary so widely even though the millicalorie threshold may be the same.

Two people may both begin to sense pain at the 220 milli-calorie level. But as this is raised three dols, one may cry out while the other will not respond at all. Both are feeling the same intensity of pain but each is handling it differently.

There is no law which fixes the level of pain that any person can bear. Not only do responses vary in the normal course of events but they can be deliberately changed in a number of ways through the use of drugs, hypnosis or conditioning. The monumental work of Pavlov showed that not only the levels of pain endurance can be changed by conditioning but the very nature of the response can be altered.

People often have an unfortunate tendency to pretend that there is something "queer" or "not quite right" about genuinely original research which suddenly upsets old and comfortable concepts. The "queerness" is compounded if the research probes into an area held sacred, such as the "soul," where "man has no business prying."

A rather large portion of the public has itself been conditioned by these attitudes to view the experiments of the Russian scientist Pavlov in this light. Granted, his research produced results which made many people feel uneasy. That was to be expected under the circumstances. After all, it must be disturbing to be shown how behavior, including our own, is determined and modified by specific mechanisms; how these mechanisms may develop and how they can be altered.

One classic experiment that is widely if not clearly known, showed that certain of our built-in reflexes, those of the involuntary nervous system over which we exercise no conscious control, can be conditioned and changed. In most hungry animals, including man, the sensory stimulation of food activates the salivary glands. Pavlov showed that by ringing a bell every time food was served to a dog, new memory-association patterns were set up that made the sound of the bell as much a sensory signal of food as the smell or sight of meat. After a while, merely the sound of a bell was enough to make a dog salivate, even though no food was present. What Pavlov had done was condition the dog's salivary reflex so that it responded to a completely different stimulus than the one provided for by nature.

The work by no means ended here. Pavlov showed that new experiences are constantly influencing the pathways and patterns of our interpretations and responses. Even the symbol of a stimulus can be made to trigger a response in the absence of the actual stimulus. This seems to be especially true of higher organisms with sufficient imagination. Dogs were conditioned to see the stick as an inflicter of pain. It became a symbol of pain and merely showing a stick to a conditioned dog was enough to set off a pain response just as though the animal were actually being beaten. This could be related to human experience where symbols, including words, often produce the same reflexive reactions as the realities they represent. A twitching finger, or even the word "tickle," can set some individuals squirming as though they actually are being tickled. And a good deal of our sexual activity is conditioned to respond to words and other symbolic stimuli.

Carrying this work even further, Pavlov was able to condition animals so that the application of one stimulus brought the response to an utterly different stimulus. The pain of an electric shock, in these animals, was not interpreted as an unpleasant threat of danger but as a promise of food. So, whenever a shock was inflicted, the animals began to salivate and show all the other signs of hunger.

Pavlov, fully aware of the impact this research would have, said: "These experiments have been apt to upset very sensitive people. But we have been able to demonstrate, though without any pretension of penetrating into the subjective world of the dog, that they are laboring under a false impression."

The possibilities opened by this work on conditioned reflexes were quickly recognized and put to planned use in many areas of training, teaching and learning. The development of conditioned responses is part of the training of astronauts, for instance. Emotional conditioning and the modification of responses to pain have gained considerable prominence in recent years. Such conditioning has become part of the training of Commando and other special combat units. It has also come into wide use in medicine and surgery, being of special benefit in painless natural childbirth.

In many otherwise normal cases, much of the pain of childbirth has been found due to the mother's attitude. Her conviction that she is about to undergo an extremely painful experience creates such anxiety, tension and fear that her pain responses become disproportionately intensified. The ordinarily bearable pain of the uterine contractions does, actually, become unbearable and some form of anesthesia is necessary.

On the other hand, the same mother could be conditioned to accept childbirth as a normally bearable experience and to regard the uterine contractions of labor as uncomfortable and perhaps mildly painful, but not agonizingly so. Such a conditioned attitude, by eliminating fear, tension and painful anticipation, serves to produce a muscular relaxation that makes possible a relatively easy, painless delivery with no or minimal anesthesia. Forms of natural childbirth have come into increasing prominence in the Soviet Union, England, France and the United States.

Possibly, in part, because of the acceptance of reflex conditioning, there has been a great resurgence of interest in hypnosis as an anesthetic technique. Like conditioning, hypnosis seems able to produce changes in patterns of interpretation and response to pain, but for more limited periods.

Because hypnosis is not effective in all areas of pain and because its mechanisms are too little known, there are as yet definite limits to its use in medical practice. Still, since it does not have the toxic or other side effects of certain drugs, it is generally considered one of the safer forms of pain relief.

The medical possibilities of hypnosis were evaluated several years ago by Dr. James Ewing, Director of Research in the Department of Psychiatry of Mercy-Douglass Hospital in Philadelphia. Under hypnosis, Dr. Ewing found, the response to pain can be modified or abolished. This involves mainly the consciousness of pain and the voluntary reaction toward it. But hypnosis, while able to diminish the reflex response to pain, such as flinching, does not eliminate it completely.

As a form of anesthesia, hypnosis was found especially useful in special types of surgery, in dentistry, childbirth and in easing the pain of ailments that have passed beyond medical help, such as terminal cancer. Hypnosis appears to have some distinct advantages in childbirth. Like natural childbirth, it eliminates the need for the anesthetic drugging which, when used excessively, has been found responsible for a high percentage of mental retardation, cerebral palsy and other brain disorders in children. Hypnosis shortens the first stages of labor, does not depress the respiration of mother or infant, raises the mother's resistance to fatigue so that she is less prone to maternal exhaustion and there is a smoother recovery after delivery.

Hypnotic anesthesia does not work in all cases. In obstetrics, it can be used alone in only twenty to twenty-five percent of selected patients. Another fifty percent will react favorably to a combination of hypnosis and drugs. In these cases there is a fifty to seventy-five percent reduction in the usual drug dose, a distinct advantage both to mother and to child.

The possibilities opened by the increasingly sophisticated use of conditioning and hypnosis reach into a number of areas. Apart from easing pain they are being used as research tools to help us explore the mechanisms of sensation, interpretation and response. Experiments with conditioned reflexes are showing how neural circuits can be altered to change natural responses or to correct unnatural responses. Hypnosis is being used to induce emotional conflicts and anxieties so that the resulting biochemical changes, with their effects on blood pressure, pain response, illness and other phenomena, can be studied.

One of the most interesting puzzles in this area of pain relief is the so-called placebo effect. The placebo is a "sugar-pill" or some similar product that is designed to have no significant physiological effect. It is the type of pill often given to hypochondriacs and where, if medication is either unwarranted or impossible, to satisfy the patient that he is being treated. The placebo is also used as a control when drugs are being tested. In such tests, some experimental subjects are given the drug and others the placebo, both of which look exactly alike so that each subject thinks he is receiving the drug. The results are sometimes surprising. Despite the fact that placebos are medically inert, they often produce a profound effect which cannot yet be explained on a physiological basis.

A wryly curious example of the placebo effect was shown in 1959 during a medical symposium under the auspices of the New York Academy of Sciences at which a new pain-relieving drug was evaluated. In a test reported by Dr. Lazlo Schwartz of Columbia University, thirty-four patients suffering from pain in the jaw were divided into two equal groups. One group was given the new drug, the other group received the placebo.

The results showed five patients clinically improved after taking the new drug. But of those receiving the placebo, six showed clinical improvement. Furthermore, those responding to placebo treatment had a better ability to open their mouths than those responding to the new drug. This was an important gain since the pain had made it extremely difficult for the patients to use their mouths.

The reasons for the placebo effect are subject to much speculation. It has been related to the mysterious easing of a toothache or other pain that sometimes takes place when we arrive in the dentist's or doctor's office. For many people, the very fact that they are receiving care, attention or concern can trigger processes which modify the mechanisms whereby pain is transmitted and felt.

Certainly we are probing more deeply than ever before into

the complicated mechanisms that determine our responses to pain. In time, this may lead us to the goal of total control whereby pain can be suppressed or abolished exactly as, when and how desired. But for the moment, among other interim advances, we have become able to appreciate the Stone Age witch doctor who, unknowingly of course, seems to have treated pain with primitive versions of all of the modern refinements from drugs and placebos to conditioning and hypnotic suggestion.

Chapter 14

THE BATTLE LINES TODAY

The sensational advances in science and technology during the last few decades have placed in man's hands incredibly potent instruments of life and death.

At no previous time in history have the implications for good or evil been so great or so clearly drawn, even if only grudgingly accepted or incompletely understood.

Most of the infectious diseases that have ravaged mankind have been brought under control or soon may be. The problems of birth, growth and aging are in the process of being solved. Virtually all the deadly plagues have been tamed and are no longer major threats to human life and health.

Equally, the struggle against pain has undergone accelerated advance and profound change. Today, the general mechanisms and pathways of pain are understood and there is growing knowledge of the biochemical and other processes involved in our responses to pain. This has made it possible for us to learn how many pain-relieving agents work, where they act and what they do. Healers need no longer blunder about in pain's dark corridors, trying this or that in the hope that something will blot out agony. Today the knowledge and techniques are approaching such precision that a specific solution can be offered for almost every particular problem.

Because we can now recognize that the pain process passes through a number of stages between the initial stimulus and the final reaction, ways have been found to attack pain in each one of these general areas.

The causes of pain can be removed. Just as the thorn that causes surface pain can be plucked out, the sources of interior pain can be treated. A muscular spasm that presses on nerves and causes pain can be relaxed with aspirin, a tranquilizer or other chemical agent. An infection can be treated in many ways and an inflammation can be reduced by a variety of drugs, old and new. In some cases, as with a ruptured appendix, surgery will serve to remove the cause of pain.

Pain can be eased or stopped by raising the thresholds of sensation and response. Such drugs as morphine, codeine and other opium derivatives are believed able to raise the pain thresholds. Chilling also seems to have this effect. On the other end of the pain pathway, the response thresholds may be raised by drugs, hypnosis and conditioning.

The pain impulses carried through the nerves can be slowed or stopped. This is nerve blocking, done by interfering with the metabolic activity that provides the nerves with the chemicals and energy needed to generate the impulses. Cocaine, novocaine and similar drugs have this effect. Since all nerves except those from the face and head pass through the spine, this main highway of the nervous system is a highly strategic center for pain relief. The fact that nerve roots from the limbs and various body areas enter the spine at known points gives spinal anesthesia a good degree of regional selectivity. It can be used to anesthetize the legs, pelvic area, abdomen and so on. There are also other ways of blocking pain by interfering with the nerve message system. One of these, chilling, or hypothermia, which slows the body's chemical processes, was used by Stone Age man and is increasingly important today. Local chilling is accomplished by spraying a small area of skin with a volatile liquid that evaporates rapidly.

Minor pains can often be eased, if not completely abolished, by focusing the attention away from the pain or by loading the nervous system with a variety of distracting sensations. People who are stimulated and excited tend to be less sensitive to pain. There are many ways of achieving this. The pain of a sore muscle can be eased by applying a counter-irritant, a liniment which stimulates other nerves with a mildly burning sensation and thus reduces the awareness of the muscular pain. In dentistry and in minor surgery, certain types of music are being used as a means of diverting the attention of the patient, increasing the message load in his nervous system and reducing the awareness of pain.

In serious surgery, where it is necessary to block out the patient's consciousness as well as all sensation, general anesthesia remains the most useful form of pain relief. Here the action is at the higher levels of the central nervous system, with the association pathways of the cerebral cortex being temporarily disrupted. As a result, sensation and motion stop; awareness, pain and the memory of the operation are eliminated. One of the more recent developments is the closed system of administration, with combinations of anesthetic inhalants and oxygen passing through a mask fitting tightly over the face. The inhaled gases pass into the blood and are carried to the brain where they shut down what amounts to the central switchboard of consciousness. Where inhalation is not possible or practical, general anesthesia can be induced rectally or by injection into the blood of one of several agents. Some barbituates are very effective in this respect.

There are certain kinds of agonizing and longlasting pain which simply cannot be relieved by any of the standard analgesic or anesthetic procedures if the patient is to remain conscious and continue to function in some way. One such condition is known as *causalgia* or burning pain. This is often caused by injury to a peripheral nerve and causes a spreading, burning pain that can become excruciatingly intensified by almost any stimulus, even contact with air, warmth, cold or dryness. In extreme cases, this is treated by surgery, cutting affected nerves so that they are no longer capable of transmitting sensation. There are also certain chemicals which can be injected to destroy nerve fibers. These must be used with extreme care so that their action is confined only to the particular nerve which is involved.

There are other forms of neurosurgery that are occasionally used to relieve great pain where other methods are not effective. One of these is called *rhizotomy,* an extremely delicate operation in which nerve roots are cut as they enter the spinal column. This is very drastic because it causes a loss of all sensation within the involved area. Another operation, perhaps more generally known, is called *leukotomy.* This is a form of brain surgery in which the white matter of the frontal lobes of the brain is cut.* This operation does not reduce the sensation or the awareness of pain. Instead it cuts the association tracts which control an individual's reaction to his environment. As a result, the patient may still feel the pain as intensely as ever before but it no longer seems to concern him.

"Yes, the pain is still there," a leukotomized person might say with characteristic passivity, "it hurts the same as always. But it doesn't bother me any more."

The six different approaches to anesthesia and analgesia that have been summarized here cover the modern battlefront against pain in the broadest general terms. There are a great number of variations as well as improvements, innovations and serious problems that are still to be solved.

The various forms of local and nerve blocking anesthesia have been improving steadily as a result of the development of new drugs, along with a more discriminating understanding of the nervous system. By blocking the synapses, or connections, of the proper nerve along a pathway, a very limited area such as a fingertip can be desensitized. Or, if necessary, larger areas can be anesthetized by blocking the pain pathways further along in the branches or in the spine roots. Where once cocaine and such a derivative as novocaine (pro-

---

* The commonly used word "lobotomy" is the general term for an operation in which brain tissue is cut.

caine) were the most effective drugs for this purpose, there has been a procession of newer, more selective and more effective agents such such as tutocaine, butyn sulfate, butesin and others. The pain-relieving range of nerve blocking anesthesia is so wide that it can cover the pulling of a tooth, the amputation of a leg or major surgery in the body's interior.

The techniques and agents used in producing general anesthesia have also been getting better as various problems have been solved. One of these problems has been a patient's sense of suffocation as he finds himself forced to inhale a gas through a mask. Almost reflexively, he would resist this type of anesthetic administration, struggling or turning his head away. This has been solved by the use of a sort of preliminary anesthesia known as induction. As the patient is brought into the operating theatre he is given an injection of sodium pentothal or a similar anesthetic drug. In less than half a minute the patient is asleep. Then, neither feeling suffocation nor struggling, the patient receives the inhalation anesthesia which continues throughout the operation.

Probably one of the major anesthetic advances in modern times, one that has saved many lives, arose out of the simple realization that the life functions of a patient have to be closely watched and controlled during an operation. Today, the anesthesiologist not only provides the proper anesthetic for the patient but also seeks to maintain his breathing, blood pressure, heart action, temperature, exchange of fluids and other functions in as closely normal a state as possible.

Throughout the ages, a serious problem of pain relief has arisen out of the fact that many of the substances used killed or damaged as often as they helped. Opium, henbane, mandrake and hemlock are toxins which can be dangerous even when used with care. The same is true of many of the modern drugs. As a result, the pharmacology of pain relief is faced with a major puzzle as well as a great challenge. Can an effective drug be found that is also safe?

Morphine is the most active alkaloid derivative of opium.

It is extremely effective and ranks as the classic drug against which other analgesics are measured. Yet, while morphine has done so much to lighten man's burden of pain, it asks a very high price. There is the matter of addiction. There is also the problem of tolerance. A person taking morphine to ease chronic pain may require a constantly increasing dosage to achieve relief. Morphine also depresses the respiratory centers, stimulates the vomiting centers, can cause severe nausea and constipation. These effects may be extremely dangerous and, in some special cases, can prove deadly. Obviously, there are many times when morphine's pain-relieving use is blocked by its possible perils.

During much of this century, chemists have been studying the molecular structure of morphine in the hope that they can rearrange it to eliminate some of its dangers. Although morphine itself was not fully synthesized until 1952, morphine-like drugs had been created earlier which were even more potent than the original. One of the early synthetics, dihydromorphinone, has a pain-relieving effect possibly five times greater than that of morphine itself and seems to have less severe gastro-intestinal side effects, but its action does not last as long and it therefore has to be given more frequently. This, in turn, increases the possibilities of tolerance and addiction.

Other morphine-like drugs have been synthesized that at first seemed very promising. These usually disappointed the early hopes for them as difficulties began to show up after continued use.

In 1939, a drug called meperidine was synthesized in Germany. This has a much simpler molecular structure than morphine and its analgesic potency is not as great. However, it is a more effective pain reliever than codeine, another opium derivative, and causes less severe respiratory and gastro-intestinal side effects than morphine. But, and this great problem still remains, it carries the risk of addiction.

Other synthetic narcotics, such as methadone, have been

created by the chemists who continue to juggle the morphine molecule in a continuing effort to find better and safer weapons against pain. So far, while a number have great value as analgesics, no way has yet been found to eliminate their dangers completely. It seems that in one way or another, drugs powerful enough to suppress severe pain, demand a price for their beneficial effect. The body is forced to adjust itself to accept these drugs and, when this is done, the body thereupon requires the drug. If the drug is then withdrawn, the body cannot readjust itself without severe consequences. This, in essence, is the nature of addiction.

At the University of Illinois College of Medicine, a study was recently made of the more powerful new analgesics by Drs. Max S. Sadove and M. J. Schriffen who reported their findings in April, 1961. Hoping to find a drug capable of easing severe visceral pain and yet not cause addiction to the drug, they tested many of the new agents but found none of them to be free from hazard.

Alphaprodine was found able to relieve intense pain for short periods. Phenazocine was useful in severe pain and also had a sedative effect. It showed good promise as an analgesic in obstetrics because it seemed easier to withdraw a patient from this drug than from more potent narcotics. The two doctors also found piminodine to be very potent and useful, especially because it causes only little respiratory depression and has a good safety factor.

The tranquilizing drugs were found to have a very useful part in pain relief. By reducing the patient's fears and tensions, these drugs make it possible to ease intense pain with smaller doses of narcotics.

Eight months after the University of Illinois study, came the report of an advance which may have far-reaching consequences—the development of an apparently non-addictive morphine substitute. The drug, with the rather complicated name of methotrimeprazine, was tested by Drs. Louis Lasagna and Thomas J. DeKornfeld of the Johns Hopkins School of

Medicine. When swallowed, the drug was not especially effective and caused side effects. But when injected, it was found to be equal to morphine in its pain-relieving effect and did not cause addiction.

This may herald a genuine breakthrough in an area which has produced as much frustration as progress. Still, experience shows that any new drug must be watched with care over a long period. Another potent drug studied by the Johns Hopkins team points up the possible perils. This agent also reduced pain without causing addiction but, as the doctors reported, "has unfortunately proved impractical for clinical use because of its bizarre mental effects."

For less intense pain, there are many non-addictive drugs, old and new, that can be used. These include such analgesics as acetylsalicylic acid (aspirin), phenacetin, phenylbutazone and others, as well as drugs being newly created or modified in the chemical laboratories. Exactly how these non-narcotic drugs work is not at all clear, although various theories exist. Some seem to raise the pain threshold, others appear to depress the perception of pain in the central nervous system. Unfortunately, these are not generally useful against the more intense pains.

Man's battlefield against pain ranges over a wide area that is constantly absorbing new forces and spreading to new combat zones. The biological and physical sciences have been drawn into the combat, as have modern technology and engineering.

The search for an effective inhalation anesthetic that has the added safety factor of not being explosive, as so many are, came to an apparently successful end late in 1961. The new anesthetic, methoxyfluorane, is non-inflammable and could be used on any anesthetic machine. According to the report by Dr. Alan Van Poznak of New York Hospital-Cornell University Medical Center, this anesthetic has been used successfully in more than 7,000 operations of all types without adverse effects that could be attributed to the drug. In some cases, patients have been anesthetized with this drug up to ten hours for protracted surgery.

At about the same time this anesthetic agent was being reported to the International Congress of Neurological Surgery in Washington, D.C., the American Chemical Society, meeting in Chicago, heard Dr. Eric R. Larsen of Midland, Michigan, describe his discovery of another non-explosive inhalation anesthetic. This is also based on a fluorine compound and is apparently potent and long lasting as well as safe.

Until the recent burst of developments coming from a number of directions, the only completely non-explosive inhalants were chloroform, nitrous oxide and trichloroethylene. But chloroform has many dangers associated with its use and the other two are not especially good anesthetics. Now, suddenly, the intensive research that has been carried on for so long is at last coming to fruition.

Music to ease pain has been used for some time without any great scientific concentration on its possibilities. Today, a greater amount of attention is being focused on this particular area of audio-analgesia. Experiments are currently under way in which music and special static sound effects, known as "white sound," are played to a patient during certain types of dental or minor surgery. Preliminary results indicate that these combinations of relaxing music and somewhat disturbing white sound crowd the thalamus and cerebral cortex with a high level of sensory input and seem to reduce the sensation and recognition of pain.

Experiments are also being conducted into the use of other forms of sensory stimulation. Visual stimuli, projections of changing colors combined with varying smells and sounds may prove to have a useful effect, but the work here is barely beginning and considerable exploratory research remains to be done.

The use of electrical stimulation is another important area of pain relief. The possibility of electricity in neuro-surgery is already proving itself, especially in the relief of the agonizing pain of terminal cancer. Dr. James C. White of Massachusetts General Hospital, the same hospital where Morton used ether in surgery, reported at the end of 1961 that he had successfully performed electrical leukotomies on a number of patients.

Dr. White, who is Professor Emeritus of Surgery at Harvard University, used the procedure in twenty-one cases of incurable cancer. He implanted small electrodes in the white matter of the frontal lobes of the brain. Then he sent electrical currents of a special radio frequency through these electrodes. Sixteen of the patients were completely relieved of pain, five had incomplete but significant relief and only one failed to benefit. What seems particularly important about this procedure is the fact that Dr. White reported no major psychological damage, one of the unfortunate and rather depressing hazards of the usual leukotomy.

Obviously, this suggests many other possible applications. There are a number of extremely painful diseases, facial neuralgia for instance, that may be relieved by this method. This could reduce or eliminate the protracted need for narcotics in those cases and thus curb the dangers of possible addiction.

All this great outpouring of discovery that has begun is just that: a bare beginning. Vast areas of pain perception and relief have only now been opened to serious exploration. But even at this early stage, the possibilities and broader implications point to a revolutionary advance toward man's ultimate understanding of man.

Chapter 15

DOORWAY INTO TOMORROW

In the span of a single lifetime the world has passed from gaslight to nuclear energy, from horse-and-wagon to space-flight, from plagues and patent medicines to immunization and antibiotics. The changes have been so vast that, although we can see them and deal with them, we still find it difficult to absorb the fact that they really happened.

It is by no means easy to accept so much so quickly. Attitudes are persistent and drag after history as a sea anchor after a storm-blown ship. We may read daily newspaper accounts of deep space probes and missions to photograph the moon and nearer planets, yet many of us still get twinges of embarrassment talking about this because we still regard it all as too fantastic to be truly real.

Here is a strange dichotomy. We have the knowledge and the technical means to make the once fantastic, commonplace and the formerly miraculous, mundane. We do this many times each day: when we turn on a light, use a telephone, take a life-essential vitamin which has been completely synthesized in a laboratory, or when we swallow a pill that will change our moods. Yet deep within many of us there persists that mixture of fear and denial of self that burdens man's achievements with inner disbelief. We often find it easier to place our faith in the inexplicable than to accept our own potential to learn, explain and achieve and to acknowledge and face our consequent responsibilities.

Nowhere does this attitude seem to penetrate more deeply than into those areas that concern man himself. Not too many centuries ago it was considered sinful to use medicine rather than faith to heal ills. Only in the last century the use of anesthesia was condemned as a violation of Divine will. Today, as science has become able to delve into man's mental and emotional processes and show that they are influenced more by chemistry and physics than by metaphysics, these aspects of the "soul" are threatened with measurability. To many, this may appear a violation of an inner refuge that was unique because it was invisible and inexplicable.

So, when we learn that the many components of sensation, interpretation, thought and behavior act through mechanisms that can be investigated, manipulated and even changed, we may tend to become uneasy; as though we have been made suddenly transparent and vulnerable. The emerging facts, therefore, become difficult to accept.

Current work on the central nervous system has entered areas fogged by clinging patches of ignorance and mysticism. What is the mechanism of learning? How, precisely, are memories stored and recalled? What are the cortical and thalamic processes that determine a response to a new experience, one for which no prior data exist in the memory cells? How are judgments formed? What is the precise nature of the chemical and electrical activity of the nerves and brain? How can the slowing of the life processes affect sensation and the response to pain?

These and similarly fundamental questions designed to explore the once taboo regions of human consciousness and reactivity are today being framed in the form of experiments. A number of answers, still tentative perhaps, have already begun to take shape.

The fact that ideas, thoughts and beliefs are intimately involved in the physiological activities of our bodies, and vice versa, has been known for some time, but the extent of this involvement has only recently become fully appreciated. A number of cases were cited by Dr. Henry K. Beecher of Harvard Medical School early in 1962 at the Second International Symposium on *Man and Civilization: Control of the Mind.*

In Australia's North Queensland not too long ago, Dr. Beecher reported, "a celebrated witch doctor 'pointed a bone' at a tribesman who at once became desperately ill and, on being examined by a competent doctor, was found to be in a dying state. The physician went to the witch doctor and told him that if he did not reverse the sickness, his own food supply would be cut off. The witch doctor leaned on the sick man's bed and told him he had not really pointed a bone at him. Recovery occurred within a few hours."

Similar events in which the biochemistry of a belief affects the total organism are common among people of all cultures, the difference being only in the beliefs which produce the effect. A middle-aged woman in the United States was found to have an inoperable cancer which would not endanger her life for some considerable time. But when a relative inadvertently told her she had cancer, she died within a few hours. In Baltimore, according to Dr. Beecher, the coroner, R. S. Fisher, has found that a number of people die each year after taking considerably less than deadly doses of poison or after inflicting relatively minor wounds upon themselves.

Apparently the biochemical changes wrought by profound convictions, fears and emotions can be as potent as the biochemical changes caused by poisons, wounds and disease. In fact, they appear able to activate the same mechanisms, albeit through different pathways. This is also true in the reverse direction, as the witch doctor's case showed. Fear may kill, but the removal of fear may also cure, as can intense emotions or beliefs if no irreversible damage has occurred. This is at the root of many seemingly miraculous cures as well as the closely related placebo effect.

Just as scientists can today manipulate the mechanisms of pain, alter its biochemistry and change its association patterns so as to make no pain at all seem like a pain in the leg, or even make an electric shock appear as a pleasant offer of food, they have begun to manipulate the mechanisms and biochemistry of fear, emotion and conviction. This has already been done for quite a number of years through such non-specific methods as hypnosis, conditioning and psychotherapy. Today, electrical and chemical therapy are increasingly being used to change the biochemistry involved in fear, anxiety, depression and other so-called mood factors that may adversely affect our health, behavior and, incidentally, our responses to pain.

The specific step-by-step changes that may take place in altering any response are often too complicated to be traced in their entirety with the means now existing. Yet, even in this apparent tangle of actions and interactions, a considerable amount of unraveling is taking place. The tranquilizing drugs which calm disturbed people and ease tensions and anxieties are also effective tools for the study of these processes, as are the newer anti-depression drugs. The actions of these chemical agents are being traced and may, ultimately, lead to the discovery of the metabolic defects that produce the original mood impairment. Considerable information has already been gathered along these lines and more is due to come.

Knowing the specific manner in which the nerves transmit their impulses of sensation and action, their "sparks of life," is extremely important to any understanding of pain and other responses. What may be a solution to this mystery was announced in November, 1960. The particular advance, whose broader implications are still difficult to measure, was the isolation of a particular protein substance which acts as a receptor of nerve impulses and helps transmit them from one nerve to another.

In order to be able to visualize the nature of this discovery, made by a group of Columbia University scientists under the leadership of Dr. David Nachmansohn, it is necessary to describe briefly what is known about the way in which a nerve impulse is transmitted.

Ordinarily, an average nerve consists of a nerve cell with its attendant fibers at each end. The fiber that carries impulses into the cell body is called the *dendron*. Usually it is short and branched, like a tree. The fiber which carries impulses out of the cell body is called the *axon*. It is usually long and slender and emerges from the side of the cell opposite to the dendron. In a nerve pathway, the cells are so arranged that the axon of one cell leads to the dendron of the next cell. The junction where these opposing fibers seem to meet is called the synapse. When an impulse travels along a nerve pathway, a stimulus is picked up by a dendron, carried into the nerve cell and then an impulse is sent out along the axon to the synapse. There the impulse stimulates the dendron of the next cell and this process is repeated all along the chain of nerves until the signal reaches its destination.

This general picture of nerve transmission was already in existence in 1940 when Dr. Nachmansohn first suggested that a particular chemical is involved in the processes that carry an impulse along a nerve. This chemical is called *acetylcholine,* ACh in biochemical shorthand.

A stimulus to a nerve end, according to this view, frees ACh which combines with a "receptor" protein in the nerve. The chemical interaction between these two substances is accompanied by an electric discharge which, in its turn, seems to stimulate the continuation of the process along the nerve path. The initial stimulus, say a pinprick or a sound, sets off the chemical action. This releases the electrical discharge which, like a spark, moves along the nerves and stimulates more chemical activity ahead of it. This, in turn, produces more electricity. When the electricity is discharged at the axon end of one nerve, a chemical stimulus reaches across the synapse and triggers the release of ACh in the dendron of the next nerve. In this way, chemistry and electricity seemingly chase each other along a chain of nerves to carry the impulse of the pinprick or the sound to the brain.

There is another chemical, according to this theory, that could shut off the chemical-electrical action at any point along the way within a few millionths of a second. This substance is *cholinesterase*, ChE, which inactivates ACh and, by thus regulating the volume of impulses moving along a nerve, protects the circuit from being overloaded. It is, in effect, an automatic circuit breaker.

This, it should be understood, was the theory developed in 1940 by Dr. Nachmansohn. It depended upon the actual presence of the "receptor" protein with which the ACh supposedly combines to generate the electrical discharge. It was this protein, never before proved to have any real existence, that was finally isolated by Dr. Seymour Ehrenpreis, one of Dr. Nachmansohn's colleagues on the Columbia University research project.

Not only does this serve to confirm the theory of how impulses are transmitted but it opens the way to a fuller understanding of how such impulses might be impeded or stopped. Certainly, it shows with a good deal of precision how various local anesthetics may act. The whole class of cocaine derivatives, including novocaine, tetracaine and the rest, has been found to combine with the receptor protein at the nerve synapses. This prevents it from reacting with acetylcholine and thus cuts off the electrical discharge essential to the propagation of the impulse and the sensation of pain.

Analysis of the protein will also open the way to the possible development of more effective and safer local anesthetics than any now available. Far beyond this, doors have been opened to the investigation of many nerve disorders as well as the still dimly-understood mechanisms whereby we sense, feel, think and respond. According to Dr. Nachmansohn, these recent discoveries are momentous and crucial. "One of the basic functions of human life is coming closer to being understood."

In the spring of 1961, some months after the Nachmansohn group reported its findings, Dr. Linus C. Pauling of the California Institute of Technology, a Nobel Laureate in chemistry, advanced a theory which could help explain the action of general anesthetics and how they produce unconsciousness.

Consciousness, we know, involves a vast number of electrical oscillations and electro-chemical interactions in the brain. These take place between electrically charged particles, or ions, and side-chains of proteins which are present in the water-like fluid which constitutes about seventy-eight percent of the brain.

The theory put forward by Dr. Pauling suggests that chloroform and similar general anesthetic agents act by causing the formation of submicroscopic crystals in the brain fluids. Since these crystals are less able to conduct electricity than the fluids themselves, the normal electrical activities of the brain are slowed to the point where unconsciousness results.

Dr. Pauling estimates that only one-tenth of one percent of the brain fluid need be converted into microcrystals to produce unconsciousness and insensitivity to pain. Support was given this theory by the laboratory demonstration that when chloroform and other such anesthetics are mixed with water, tiny crystals such as those envisioned in the brain do actually form. Further support comes from the fact that when the brain is cooled ten or fifteen degrees, similar crystals form and unconsciousness is produced even in the absence of anesthetics.

The manner in which the anesthetics form the microcrystals is explained in the following way: The molecules of anesthetic fit into the spaces that separate small groups of water molecules, enclosing them and reducing their motion. This stabilizes the water molecules, reduces their molecular heat and allows them to crystallize.

This theory opens a whole new realm of speculation regarding events and factors that may affect the electrical activity involved in thought, sensation, emotion, muscular function and the other processes of life. It may also make possible a new approach to anesthesia, in which anesthetics are tailor-made so that their molecular size and structure are best suited to stabilize the molecules of brain fluid and produce unconsciousness.

One of the newest forms of anesthesia which seems to hold

considerable promise for the future is achieved by sending an electric current through the head of the patient. This seems to produce none of the disorientation or other after-effects of earlier types of general anesthesia.

The announcement of electrical anesthesia came in September, 1961, from Lt. General Arthur G. Trudeau of the United States Army. The experiments had been conducted by a medical team at the University of Mississippi Medical School. Two electrodes were fastened to the patient's temples and through these passed a current coming from an oscillator and amplifier. As the current was turned on, the patient seemed to fall asleep within a matter of seconds and the operation could begin. The patient remained asleep so long as the current was on. When the operation was completed, the electricity was turned off and the patient awoke in a few seconds.

A later report on this method was made by Dr. M. Don Turner of the University of Mississippi after it had been used on nineteen patients including fourteen advanced surgical risks. The operations lasted from twenty minutes to two and a half hours. Absolutely no brain damage was reported as a result of this anesthesia. Yet some unusual effects did turn up, according to Dr. Turner. "At least three of the patients were fully aware during surgery although they felt no pain. Three other patients, in retrospect, also reported feeling discomfort at some point. We do not know why some subjects do not have total amnesia."

This work is quite different from the electrical leukotomies performed by Dr. James C. White. But both represent a completely new approach to pain relief and anesthesia, probably the first really basic change in more than a century. The precise way in which the current acts and its effects upon the electro-chemistry of the brain are yet to be determined. But, even as an experimental technique, it opens a new and highly promising pathway for investigation into the cortical mechanisms of pain and consciousness.

Still another area of pain relief, one involving the very basic activities of life, is hypothermia, the lowering of the body temperature. Chilling has been used from earliest times to relieve pain but it is only in recent years that this process has received a concentration of scientific attention. Although its potential is still far from fully developed, this technique has already caused a revolution in surgery, pain relief and a number of other areas of life and death.

Heat, as we know, is an essential component of all activity, including the biochemical and bioelectrical activity of life. The speed of chemical reactions increases as heat increases, decreases as temperature falls. In the adult human, the life processes are designed to function most effectively at an average internal temperature of about 98.6 degrees Fahrenheit. If the interior body temperature falls, the body's chemical processes slow, and the needs of the cells for oxygen and other substances essential to metabolic activity decline. The heartbeat slows, the flow of blood slows, the speed of the nerve impulses slows. Even the sensitive brain cells, which quickly suffer destructive damage if they are briefly deprived of oxygen and blood at normal temperatures, can survive undamaged for relatively long periods of time in the hypothermic state.

The controlled cooling of the human body that produces hypothermia, or refrigeration anesthesia, is made possible by a number of methods. The temperature may be reduced by packing the body with ice, wrapping it in cooling blankets, by pumping chilled blood into the system or by inserting a refrigerating element into a large blood vessel. The process must be carefully controlled at all stages in order to prevent any tissue-damaging freezing. Great care must also be taken when restoring the body temperature to normal after the operation.

Since this form of anesthesia slows the life processes and reduces the need of the cells and organs for blood and oxygen, previously impossible forms of surgery have been made almost commonplace. Using an artificial heart and artificial lungs in conjunction with hypothermia makes it possible to shunt blood around these organs. In 1959, British surgeons used such a technique to perform an operation that required about forty-five minutes of work on a relatively dry and empty heart. The patient's temperature was reduced to 59°F. and the operation was successfully completed.

Similar operations have been performed here and in other parts of the world. In 1961, Professor C. Kolesnikov, director of the Institute of Cardiovascular Surgery in Moscow, reported twenty successful open-heart operations upon patients whose body temperatures had been reduced to as low as 50°F. And at Duke University School of Medicine, Dr. W. C. Sealy and a team of surgeons were able to perform a remarkably delicate brain operation by reducing the temperature of the patient to 41°F, only nine degrees above freezing.

A technique of limited hypothermia that may prove highly useful was announced in October, 1961, by Dr. Irving S. Cooper of St. Barnabas Hospital of Chronic Diseases in New York. Instead of lowering the temperature of the whole body and thus slowing all of the life processes of the patient, liquid nitrogen is used to freeze only small areas of the brain, blocking the activity of the nerves which conduct pain data. This form of refrigeration anesthesia is quite new and awaits more work before its possibilities can be evaluated.

From an experimental standpoint, hypothermia is far more than a remarkable anesthetic that can allow a surgeon the time required to perform complicated operations upon delicate organs. Scientists have come to recognize it as an invaluable research tool which may help them dispel a number of the mysteries that still obsure the processes of life, aging and death.

Exceptional exploratory research has shown that even humans can be chilled to the point where the heartbeat and breathing stop and what amounts to physiological death sets in, then be restored to life. In these cases, the temperature is too low to sustain the biochemical and bioelectrical activities of the organism as a whole and the organs thereupon cease functioning. But certain life processes within each separate cell continue at a very slow rate, keeping the individual cells alive. Such a body, while physiologically dead and no longer operating as an organized structure, still retains life in the biological sense.

In two recently recorded cases, men who had accidentally been rapidly frozen and were physiologically dead for several hours were restored to normal life. One of these "returns from death" took place in Northern India and was reported last year in the *Indian Journal of Public Health* (Volume 5, No. 3). The other occurred in the Soviet Union on March 26, 1960 and was reported in *Science and Life* (1961, No. 4).

In both cases the men involved had no heartbeat, no pulse, no breathing. Their eyes were open and frosted over and the pupils did not react to light. The bodies were stiff and gave off a "hollow" or "wooden" sound when hammered upon. Furthermore, they had apparently been in this state for several hours when resuscitation procedures were begun. Ordinarily, both of these men would have been pronounced as unquestionably dead and their bodies disposed of. Yet both of them are alive and at work today.

In such extreme hypothermic states, the physiologically dead body can theoretically remain biologically alive and restorable for an indefinite period. During that time, sensation stops, the heart and circulation stop, breathing and the activity of the body organs cease, the aging process seems to come to a halt. The body is dead in virtually all respects save one, the cells do not decompose or undergo irreversible changes. What is more, tests by Dr. Stanley W. Jacob and J. E. Dunphey of the University of Oregon Medical School have shown that certain human cells, including spermatozoa, can survive at a temperature of 1° Absolute, or 458.6° below zero, Fahrenheit. This does not imply that a whole human body can be kept at that temperature and then restored. But it does indicate that the possibilities inherent in hypothermia reach into the realm of what we now deem fantasy.

Researchers are investigating the use of hypothermia to reduce metabolic stress and allow gravely ill or badly damaged bodies a better chance to repair themselves. Such work, under way in the United States, Great Britain, France, the Soviet Union, China and other countries, has already produced some extremely encouraging results. In Baltimore, Drs. John M. Allen and James Estes of University Hospital reported dramatic success resulting from the use of long hypothermia on five patients dying of septic shock. The patients were all suffering from massive infections due to various causes and had failed to respond to all other treatment. They were on the verge of death when hypothermia was induced and maintained for periods ranging from fifty-one hours to twenty-one days. Four of the patients, who would otherwise have been dead, recovered completely. The fifth died of a complication not related to the hypothermia.

This use of artificial hibernation, still in a dawning state of experiment, has successfully been applied in the Soviet Union and other countries to prevent brain damage to newborn infants suffering from asphyxiation, is being used in attempts to slow and perhaps reverse damage to kidneys, heart and other organs.

Meanwhile scientists in an entirely different area of investigation are designing experiments to test the feasibility of using hypothermia to allow the human exploration of deep space. Only some such form of suspended animation, it is believed, will make it possible for us to bridge the vast gulfs of space, time and loneliness that separate us from the distant planets and the stars.

Man has indeed come a long way from the savage who first discovered the pain-relieving properties of cold. The scientific hypothermia into which this ancient discovery evolved has now provided us with a research instrument with which to investigate and even manipulate some of the fundamental processes of life. Similar developments are taking place with electricity and molecular chemistry.

The possibilities lend themselves to interesting speculation. Knowledge seems to have a disconcerting way of leading to increasing complexity rather than simplicity. Once pain was a simple matter of demons. It could be banished by driving the demons away. Thousands of years of thought, investigation and science have shown us that no phenomenon is single and simple, but that all events are somehow related and exercise an effect upon one another. This leads to another thought; that the simplicity of the primitive was apparent, not real. It fragmented the universe into an infinity of separate and unrelated events. This is complexity in its anarchic extreme. Knowledge, on the other hand, relates and binds. The apparent complexity it brings is, in effect, a growing order of unity.

Where man began to fight pain by chasing demons, he today has come to understand that pain is intimately involved with the mechanisms and processes of life itself. And in his struggle to conquer pain he has come to a closer knowledge of himself, what he is and how he functions.

Most useless pain has already been conquered. Techniques are available for dealing with virtually all pain, and these are being constantly improved. The day may not be far when pain, as such, is no longer a problem. But the questions of human awareness and responsiveness will take longer to solve.

The human brain, through which we know all pain and knowledge, weighs but three pounds yet it controls, regulates and integrates all of our life processes as well as how we feel, think, act and respond. During an average second of its activity it performs about five trillion operations, each signaled by an electro-chemical discharge.

Here, in charting, integrating, analysing and understanding even one second's activity of the brain, lies the ultimate adventure. When that can be done, and it is not beyond the scope of the human brain ultimately to understand itself, man's conquest of pain will be complete.

Selected Bibliography

Selected Bibliography

SELECTED BIBLIOGRAPHY

Atkinson, D. T., *Magic, Myth and Medicine*, World, New York, 1956.

Bankoff, G., *The Conquest of Pain*, Macdonald, London, 1946.

Bass, A. D., and Brodie, B. B. (ed.), *The Evolution of Nervous Control*, American Association for the Advancement of Science, Washington, 1959.

Bernal, J. D., *Science in History*, Cameron Assoc., New York, 1957.

Best, C. H., and Taylor, N. B., *Physiological Basis of Medical Practice*, Williams & Wilkins, Baltimore, 1950.

Best, C. H., and Taylor, N. B., *The Human Body*, Holt, New York, 1956.

Breasted, J. H., *The Edwin Smith Surgical Papyrus*, University of Chicago Press, Chicago, 1930.

Brim, C. J., *Medicine in the Bible*, Froben, New York, 1936.

Browne, E. G., *Arabian Medicine*, Cambridge University Press, Cambridge, 1921.

Burroughs Wellcome Co., *Anesthetics, Ancient and Modern*, London, 1907.

California Medicine (vol. 86), *Symposium on Pain*, San Francisco, 1957.

Camac, C. N. B., *From Imhotep to Harvey*, Hoeber, New York, 1931.

Castiglione, A. (E. B. Krumbhaar, ed.), *A History of Medicine*, Knopf, New York, 1958.

Castiglione, A., *The Renaissance of Medicine in Italy*, Johns Hopkins Press, Baltimore, 1934.

CIBA Symposia, *Medicine in Ancient Egypt*, Vol. 1, No. 10, January, 1940.

Dampier, W. C., *A History of Science*, Cambridge University Press, Cambridge, 1944.

Ebbell, B. (trans.), *The Papyrus Ebers*, Milford, London, 1937.

Elliotson, J., *Numerous Cases of Surgical Operations Without Pain in the Mesmeric State*, Ballière, London, 1843.

Ellis, E. S., *Ancient Anodyna and Primitive Anesthesia*, Heinemann, London, 1946.

Frazer, J. G., *The Golden Bough*, Macmillan, London, 1910.

Friedenwald, H., *The Jews and Medicine*, Johns Hopkins Press, Baltimore, 1944.

Fülop-Miller, R., *Triumph Over Pain*, Bobbs-Merrill, New York, 1938.

Gordon, B. L., *The Romance of Medicine*, Davis, Philadelphia, 1944.

Haggard, W. H., *Mystery, Magic and Medicine*, Doubleday, New York, 1933.

Jayne, W. A., *Healing Gods of Ancient Civilization*, Yale University Press, New Haven, 1925.

Journal of Chronic Diseases (vol. 4, No. 1), *Symposium on Pain and Its Relief*, St. Louis, 1956.

Keele, K. D., *The Anatomies of Pain*, Blackwell, Oxford, 1957.

Keys, T. E., *The History of Surgical Anesthesia*, Schuman, New York, 1945.

Lubbock, J., *The Origins of Civilization and the Primitive Condition of Man*, Longman's, London, 1911.

Morse, W. R., *Chinese Medicine*, Hoeber, New York, 1914.

Muthu, D. C., *The Antiquity of Hindu Medicine and Civilization*, Hoeber, New York, 1931.

Newall, C. F., *The Problem of Pain in Nature*, Paisley, London, 1917.

Ogilvie, H., and Thomson, W. A. H. (ed.), *Pain and Its Problems*, Eyre & Spottiswoode, London, 1950.

Poynter, F. N. L. (ed.), *The Brain and Its Functions*, Blackwell, Oxford, 1958.

Riesman, D., *The Story of Medicine in the Middle Ages*, Hoeber, New York, 1935.

Robinson, V., *Victory over Pain*, Schuman, New York, 1946.

Seeman, B., *The River of Life*, Norton, New York, 1961.

Sigerist, H. E., *The Great Doctors*, Norton, New York, 1938.

Simpson, J. Y., *Answer to Religious Objections Advanced Against the Employment of Anesthetic Agents in Midwifery and Surgery*, Sutherland & Knox, Edinburgh, 1847.

Simpson, M. W. H., *Arab Medicine and Surgery*, Oxford University Press, London, 1922.

Singer, C. J., *Greek Biology and Greek Medicine,* Oxford University Press, London, 1922.

Susruta (trans. by Hoernle, A. F. R.), *Susruta-Samhita,* Calcutta, 1897.

Thorndike, L. A., *A History of Magic and Experimental Science,* Macmillan, New York, 1941.

Walsh, J. J., *Medieval Medicine,* Macmillan, New York, 1920.

Woolmer, R., *The Conquest of Pain,* Knopf, New York, 1961.

Bibliography

Index

INDEX

BERNARD SEEMAN

gave up a professional career as a metallurgical chemist to devote full time to writing. He has been medical and science editor for *Magazine Digest, Journal of Living,* and *People Today,* and his articles have appeared in many national magazines, including the *Saturday Evening Post, N. Y. Times Magazine, Pageant, Holiday, American Mercury, Better Homes & Gardens, Today's Health, Family Circle,* and others. His books include *How To Live with Diabetes,* which he co-authored with Henry Dolger, M.D., and the recently published study of blood, *The River of Life.*

Mr. Seeman is a member of the Federation of American Scientists, the Association for the Advancement of Science, the Academy of Political Science, and the National Academy of Recording Arts and Sciences.